FOOD: NEED, GREED & MYOPIA

Exploitation and Starvation in a World of Plenty

Geoffrey Yates

'There is enough for every man's need but not for every man's greed'
Mahatma Ghandi

Earthright Publications

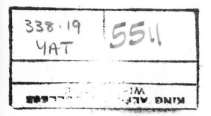
British Library Cataloguing in Publication Data
Yates, Geoffrey
    Food : need, greed & myopia : exploitation
    and starvation in a world of plenty.—
    2nd ed., fully rev.
    I. Food industry and trade
    I. Title
    338.I'9   HD9000.5

    ISBN 0-907367-04-6

First published in 1980
2nd edition, fully revised, 1986

Published by Earthright Publications,
8 Ivy Avenue, Ryton, Tyne and Wear, NE40 3PU

Printed by Tyneside Free Press Ltd, Newcastle upon Tyne
on recycled paper from PaperBack Ltd, London

ISBN 0 907367 04 6

FOREWORD

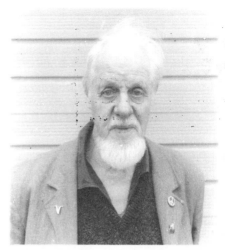

Geoffrey Yates is a retired school-teacher in his eighties and this is a second, completely revised, edition of his first book, *FOOD: NEED, GREED AND MYOPIA*, published in 1980.

He first started practising vegetarianism in the 1930s. He was uneasy about eating meat, though at the time he wasn't clear why — a mixture of cruelty and ecological factors, he remembers.

It was not until he retired from teaching physics in 1960 that he had the time to develop his interest in the whole complex issue of food. He was already a member of the Vegetarian Society and after he retired Geoff became a member of the Conservation Society's food study group. Later he joined the World Development Movement and Tyneside Friends of the Earth (FoE), again concentrating his attention on the food issue.

When FoE set up a series of Workers' Educational Association seminars in Newcastle on the world food problem, Geoff prepared one of the lectures. This, with further notes, formed the basis of the first edition of *FOOD: NEED, GREED AND MYOPIA*. He admits it is a personal view but feels that it is a view towards which society is moving.

The second edition is much expanded — the result of several years more reading. Most sections have been completely updated and rewritten and much of the section on growth and economics is new. The book has many new illustrations and the updated booklist and lists of periodicals and organizations provide sources of further information.

CONTENTS

TABLES AND DIAGRAMS

ACKNOWLEDGEMENTS

I would like again to gratefully acknowledge the advice and valuable suggestions for improving the text, of Mrs Kathleen Jannaway of the Movement for Compassionate Living and Dr Alan Long of the Vegetarian Society. My thanks are also due to Mrs Annie Lockwood and Miss Monica Frisch who have worked hard on successive revisions and extensions of the original text. Monica has undertaken the laborious task of typing and retyping the script, collecting, updating and extending statistical and other data required, and much other hard work involved.

Acknowledgements are also due to Clare Brannen for preparing most of the diagrams and the drawings on pages 30, 54 and 78, Mary Morris for some of the diagrams from the first edition, Christopher Beaton for the cartoon on page 60, Jean Plantu for the cartoon on the back cover, Andes Press Agency for the photographs on the cover and page 6, Annie Lockwood for the photo of the author, Format Photographers for the photo on page 4, Fewsters Agricultural Services Ltd for the photo on page 6, Monica Frisch for the photomontage on page 46, Compassion in World Farming for the photo on page 76, *New Internationalist* for permission to use the table on page 2, *The Sunday Times* for the extract on page 5, *New Socialist*, the monthly left magazine for the extract on page 5, *Oxfam News* for the extract on page 28, and Elizabeth Cook for the index.

The cover photograph by Carlos Reyes shows a woman in Sudan tending melons grown alongside dura, a kind of sorghum.

I INTRODUCTION

"Every two seconds of this year a child will die of hunger or disease. And no statistic can express what it is like to see even one child die . . . to see the uncomprehending panic in eyes which are still the clear and lucid eyes of a child."

"There is already a deteriorating food situation in Africa: food production not keeping pace with population growth, and growing dependence on food imports."*

Common Crisis: The Second Brandt Report

About 570 million people are undernourished, 800 million are illiterate, 1,500 million have little or no access to medical services, 250 million do not go to school, and 15 million children die annually (about one child every two seconds) either from starvation or illness due to undernourishment — according to World Bank estimates. Yet the world could and indeed does produce more than enough to feed all its human population.

The world's total cereal crop (wheat, rice, barley, maize, millet and sorghum) was 1,650 million tonnes in 1981 and had increased at an average rate of 2.7% per annum over the previous decade. This means the world produces about one kilogram of grain per day for every man, woman and child on earth (i.e. about 3,000 calories — more than is necessary — and adequate protein). The world also produces 300 grammes per person per day of root crops, and large quantities of other foods. There is no clear reason why people should starve to death — but they continue to do so.

The direct human consumption of grain in the United Kingdom is under 200 grammes per head per day, plus some grain used for beer and other products. We grow the equivalent of 700—900 grammes of grain per head per day but the bulk of it is of animal fodder quality only, and we import some of the wheat used for bread making. Of course land used to grow fodder wheat for animals could be used to produce a somewhat smaller quantity of higher protein wheat for human use; and if we grew such wheat for human consumption only, a much smaller acreage would suffice. A considerably reduced number of food animals could revert to living mainly by grazing This would avoid much environmental damage and cost very much less in food subsidies, but it would reduce outputs of meat and dairy produce.

This does not however provide an answer to the question of why people starve in a world of potential plenty for all. One clue to the answer is that in poor countries people can starve in areas where good land is left unused. Richard Body in *Farming in the Clouds* describes an area in Senegal (West Africa) near the Senegal River where hundreds of thousands of hectares of rich alluvial silt, first rate land, go largely uncultivated except for some 4,000 hectares which grow sugar and tomatoes to be sent to the capital, Dakar. Yet on this same land there are children with the now all too familiar extreme nutrition deficiency symptoms, swollen bellies and emaciated limbs, while

* The second quotation above from *Common Crisis*, while a statement of fact, is misleading in attributing Africa's need for food imports merely to population growth.

their mothers looked prematurely aged. This is not an isolated example. People who lack purchasing power can starve to death in a country with great reserves of cultivatable but uncultivated land (SEE 'How may people could the world feed?'). Another clue to the answer is 'cash crops' (SEE later).

TABLE I: CALORIE INTAKES

Calories are units of the energy provided by food; proteins are the ingredients of food involved in tissue growth and repair. Both are necessary, especially for growing children (SEE section on nutrition). Generally enough calories means also enough protein but by no means always.

Lowest calorie intake per day, 1983			Highest calorie intake per day, 1983		
Country	Calorie intake per head/day	% of needs	Country	Calorie intake per head/day	% of needs
1. Ghana	1,573	68	1. Ireland	4,054	162
2. Chad	1,620	68	2. Denmark	4,023	150
3. Mali	1,731	74	3. East Germany	3,787	145
4. Kampuchea	1,792	81	4. Belgium	3,743	142
5. Uganda	1,807	78	5. Bulgaria	3,711	148
6. Mozambique	1,844	79	6. Yugoslavia	3,642	143
7. Burkina Faso	1,879	79	7. USA	3,616	137
8. Haiti	1,903	84	8. Czechoslovakia	3,613	146
9. Bangladesh	1,922	83	9. UA Emirates	3,591	n.a.
10. Guinea	1,987	86	10. Libya	3,581	152
11. Laos	1,992	90	11. France	3,572	142
12. Vietnam	2,017	93	12. Holland	3,563	133
13. Nepal	2,018	86	13. Greece	3,554	142
14. Angola	2,041	87	14. New Zealand	3,549	134
15. India	2,047	93	15. Austria	3,524	134
16. Sierra Leone	2,049	85	16. Italy	3,520	140
17. Zambia	2,054	89	17. Hungary	3,520	134
18. Kenya	2,056	88	18. Switzerland	3,451	128
19. El Salvador	2,060	90	19. Canada	3,428	129
20. Ecuador	2,072	91	20. Kuwait	3,423	n.a.
30. Ethiopia	2,162	93	27. UK	3,232	128
39. Sudan	2,250	96	30. Australia	3,189	120
60. China	2,562	109	41. Cuba	2,997	130

The estimate of a person's calorie requirement per day varies from country to country according to the FAO/WHO assessment of the age make-up of the population. Children need fewer calories (they need more per body weight than adults but are much lighter). Since there are proportionately many more children in developing countries, this leads to a wide difference in the national average requirement. The lowest of these in 1983 was Benin with 2,133 and the highest Switzerland with 2,696. These are average figures — just as there are people on the breadline in Ireland, there are those who have enough to eat in Chad.

Source: World Bank, World Development Report 1985, via *New Internationalist*

Up to 600 million young children in the developing world may be suffering from dietary deficiency — the consequences of this may be mental as well as physical damage. Lack of food can produce marasmus. The child victim of this disease is like a skeleton covered by skin. It results from simple starvation or debilitating illness. The child victim of kwashiorkor, by contrast does not look thin. This malignant form of malnutrition results in an enlarged abdomen and a tight skin swollen with retained water. The diet here lacks protein and often other nutrients, but they are getting some food. Apart from these wasting diseases, undernourishment weakens the body's resistance to other illnesses. While this is so in the developing nations, citizens of highly developed countries suffer from the avoidable results of over-eating: obesity, indigestion, constipation, heart disease etc.

While official development aid amounts to some £14 billion* a year the world's military expenditure is around £300 billion per year and while money is being spent on more nuclear weapons the world already has a nuclear bomb stockpile of 50,000, with a destructive power of 700,000 Hiroshimas, enough to extinguish all life on earth, several times over!

That 20 times as much is being spent on potential destruction as is being employed to relieve human misery highlights the problem.

In the world today, one person's greed is another person's need — of course a few gluttons cannot produce a famine but 1,000 million consuming in effect many times too much, (and not only of food), will inevitably produce want elsewhere. The all but ubiquitous myopic (or 'blind spot') vision of mankind, prevents such facts being clearly seen and acknowledged.

MYOPIA OR TUNNEL VISION

We see only what we want to see. Nelson deliberately avoided seeing the signal to retreat which he intended to disregard by putting the telescope to his blind eye. When some of Captain Cook's crew went ashore at a South Sea island, the natives showed great interest in the rowing boats in which they came, but ignored the large ship itself, anchored some distance off shore, though it was clearly visible. They too had rowing boats but a large sailing ship was beyond their 'apperceptive range'. Whether deliberately, subconsciously or otherwise, people tend to avoid seeing what is beyond their scope, disturbing or unwanted. Thus economists and politicians ignore the wastefulness of consumption-oriented, competitive market economics. Abstraction has its own form of myopia, or 'ignore-ence' (the capacity to ignore) which is quite unlike ignorance (lack of knowledge), and differs again from deliberate evasion, or pretence, or plain lying (of which there is no shortage today in sundry places).

The human mind has a capacity for failing to see the obvious and for holding on to obviously harmful and obsolete ideas and values — a form of mental myopia, blind spot vision — combined with a powerful capacity of self-deception and ability to ignore (ignore-ence). Barbara Ward spoke of 'tunnel vision' — the rich nations suffer from this 'tunnel vision': like the elephants round a water hole they do not notice the other animals. It hardly enters their minds that they are trampling the place to pieces. Ronald Higgins in The Seventh Enemy calls it 'individual blindness' (which with 'political inertia' constitutes the 'seventh enemy' — there being six others). This mental capacity is easier to illustrate than to define.

*NOTE Throughout this book 1 billion = 1,000 million

Two incidents from an article in the *Sunday Times* (15th January 1984) illustrate this kind of mental blindness; the article by John Carey reflects on his experience of teaching English Literature in India.

(a) He was talking to a young Indian lecturer who said 'it is hard for us to imagine the slum conditions described in Victorian novels'; and went on to suggest that the British Council might aid understanding by sending out 'illustrative material'. John Carey remarks that he just looked around. 'All around the university perimeter on the dirty sidewalks were neat piles of cooking untensils, belonging to pavement dwelling families. The grown-ups were off doing casual labour. The toddlers could be seen, playing almost naked on muck heaps. Slightly older children were patiently sorting piles of plastic bags, rags and bottles for resale. Krool, the rag and bone dealer from *Bleak House* would have been quite at home'.

(b) He describes how he was driven along at 100 kilometres per hour by a young doctor along a country road, blaring on his horn, and scattering bedraggled peasant women and children, trudging along the dusty verges, while he joked with an Indian professor about their alarm. At their destination, a wild life park, the young doctor spoke seriously of the need to conserve crocodiles.

One can only conclude that some upper class Indians find it easier to identify with characters in novels while they see their own peasants and their own poor as inferior animals.

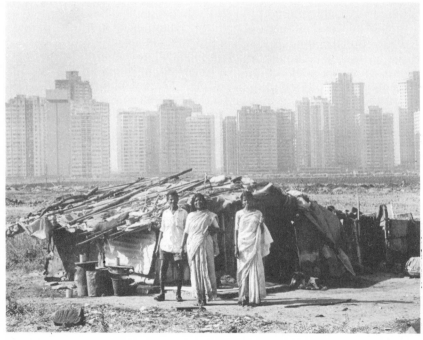

Maggie Murray/Format

Ronald Higgins in *The Seventh Enemy* gave many instances of 'individual blindness'. The Vietnam War and the slaughter by American troops of Vietnamese civilians, including women and children as at My Lai in 1967: the trial of Lieutenant Calley shocked many Americans for a while, but after Calley's conviction the mail was 100 to 1 against the verdict, according to the White House. There is nothing peculiar to America in this outlook. All nations resort to absurd rationalisations like 'the defence of liberty' to justify anything, for example incinerating a city by high density bombing. The cool attitude of many Germans to the wartime concentration camps and the massacre of Jews is another example.

Apart from this myopia, there is the 'double voice' aspect of established power. For example, the public and more private voices of the United States:

Public:

'The international purposes of the United States in the late twentieth century are co-operation, not hegemony or domination; partnership not confrontation; a decent life for all not exploitation.'

Report of the National Bipartisan (Kissinger) Commission on Central America, 1984

'As I flew back this evening, I had many thoughts. In just a few days families across America will gather to celebrate Thanksgiving. And again, as our forefathers who voyaged to America, we travelled to Geneva with peace as our goal and freedom as our guide. For there can be no greater good than the quest for peace — and no finer purpose than the preservation of freedom.'

Ronald Reagan to Congress, 21st Nov. 1985

More private:

'... we have about 50 per cent of the world's wealth, but only 6.3 per cent of its population ... in this situation we cannot fail to be the object of envy and resentment. Our real task in the coming period is to devise a pattern of relationships which will permit us to maintain this position of disparity without detriment to our national security ... our attention will have to be concentrated everywhere on our immediate national objectives. We need not deceive ourselves that we can afford today the luxury of altruism and world benefaction ... we should cease to talk about vague — and for the Far East — unreal objectives such as human rights, the raising of the living standards and democratisation. The day is not far off when we are going to have to deal in straight power concepts. The less we are hampered by idealistic slogans the better.'

George Kennan's Policy Planning Study, 23rd February 1948.

Source: 'The Evil Empire' by Noam Chomsky, *New Socialist* January 1986

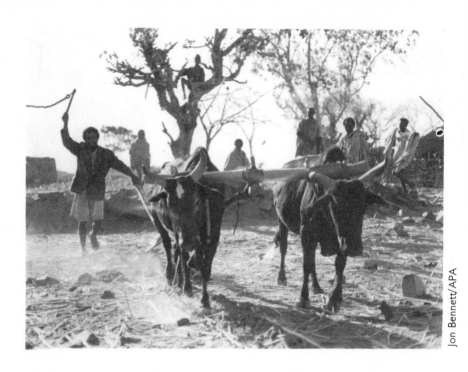

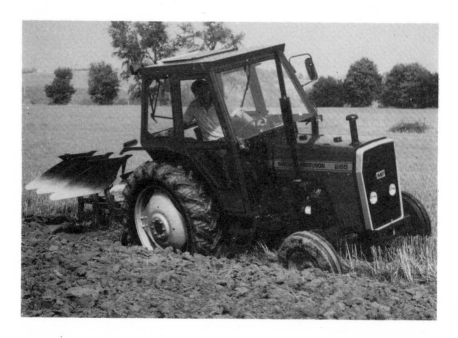

2 THE WORLD FOOD PROBLEM
WORLD FOOD PRODUCTION

Vegetable foods (plants) are the basis of all animal life and humans are, and always have been, mainly vegetable eaters. Grain crops are, and for the last ten millenia probably have been, the most significant item involved as Table 2 shows. Grain crops today provide directly more than 50% of the world's protein and energy needs. If their contribution to meat, dairy produce and alcohol are added they provide 75% of human protein and energy needs; although this additional 25% used over 40% of the total grain crop.

The world produces about 1,650 million tonnes of food and feed grains annually and the rich industrialized world consumes half, although it contains only about a quarter of the world's population. Over 40% of the world's cereal harvest is fed to livestock, mainly in the rich industrialized 'North'. In the poorer countries most of the cereal crop is consumed directly, in Britain and Western Europe 30%, and in North America only 14%. These figures highlight the huge differences in wealth between the richer and poorer countries of the world. They are, of course, averages and averages are deceptive, especially in the poorer countries since there are really no completely poor countries, only some with a much larger proportion of impoverished people.

TABLE 2: MAJOR WORLD FOOD CROPS

Top seven crops (million tonnes)

Wheat	500	Barley	167
Rice	448	Cassava	126
Maize	415	Sweet potato	113
Potato	295		

Crops produced in excess of 10 million tonnes per year

Sugar	113	Cottonseed	30
Soybean	87	Water melon	26
Grapes	68	Yam	25
Sorghum	66	Onions	23
Tomato	56	Plantains	20
Oats	44	Groundnuts	19
Banana	41	Sunflower seed	16
Apples	40	Rapeseed	15
Oranges	38	Beans	15
Cabbage	37	Mango	14
Coconut	34	Cucumbers & gherkins	12
Rye	32	Carrots	11
Millets	31	Peas	10

Figures are the average of production for 1982, 1983 and 1984

Source: FAO

FIGURE I: WORLD MEAT PRODUCTION (1984)

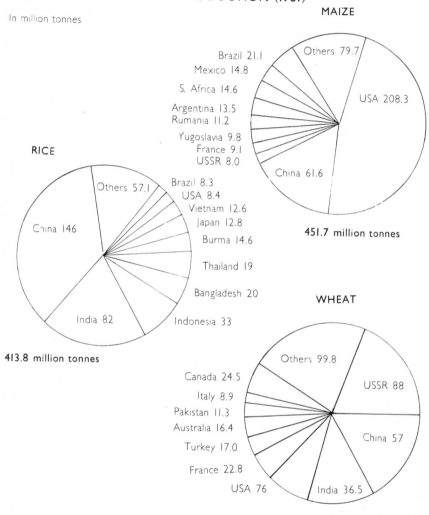

Pork
55.5 million tonnes
Total: 137.2 million tonnes

Beef
45.7 million tonnes

Poultry   Lamb
29.9 million tonnes 6.1 million
                      tonnes

Source: FAO

FIGURE 2: WORLD CEREAL PRODUCTION (1981)

In million tonnes

MAIZE

Brazil 21.1
Mexico 14.8
S. Africa 14.6
Argentina 13.5
Rumania 11.2
Yugoslavia 9.8
France 9.1
USSR 8.0

Others 79.7
USA 208.3
China 61.6

451.7 million tonnes

RICE

Others 57.1
China 146
India 82

Brazil 8.3
USA 8.4
Vietnam 12.6
Japan 12.8
Burma 14.6
Thailand 19
Bangladesh 20
Indonesia 33

413.8 million tonnes

WHEAT

Others 99.8
Canada 24.5
Italy 8.9
Pakistan 11.3
Australia 16.4
Turkey 17.0
France 22.8
USA 76

USSR 88
China 57
India 36.5

458.2 million tonnes

THE GREEN REVOLUTION

In the two decades between about 1950 and 1970 grain production per hectare in the highly developed world doubled; in America it trebled. It was mainly due to genetic seed improvements and of course extensive use of fertilizers and pesticides.

It had much less beneficial effect, at least initially, in the developing world where the capital to purchase fertilizers etc. is frequently lacking; it has thus tended to accentuate unequal distribution of land there, by eliminating the smaller, poorer, landowner. The benefit of many innovations in the Third World is neutralized or even reversed by intense poverty, rapid population increases, and the use of some of the best land, which could produce food for local consumption, for cash crops; in some areas also by continuous drought and the spread of deserts (due to use of trees for fuel and overgrazing of sparse grass land). Loan repayments and other handicaps produced by high finance also are involved.

'In Colombia malnutrition is common but fertile land is used to grow 18 million dollars worth of cut flowers for the rich world.

In the Sahel even during the great drought of 1974, export productions like peanuts from Mali actually increased while tens of thousands starved.'

Econews January 1980

CAUSES OF THE WORLD FOOD PROBLEM

Since, with very rare exceptions, only poor people die of starvation or suffer from severe malnutrition, the immediate cause is poverty.

Poverty results from or is greatly aggravated by

(1) rapid population expansion
(2) the extremely inequable distribution of wealth between rich and poor countries and also between individuals in both
(3) the human exploitation
   a)   of other humans, e.g. slavery
   b)   of animals, e.g. intensive factory farming, and
   c)   of the environment e.g. deforestation
4)   the harmful effects of false ideas, notions and mental outlooks. These can be commonly accepted prejudices or the result of propaganda.

These are of course interconnected and there are also other aspects of the problem; while the food problem itself is only the most stark aspect of the whole problem of exploitation and deprivation.

THE POPULATION EXPLOSION

The world food problem has been greatly aggravated by the rapid population growth, especially in the poorer world. It persists because of the social, economic, financial, and political constitution of contemporary society.

In itself it need not produce poverty. The population expansion has been so rapid recently that it has been called the 'population explosion'.

At the dawn of the agricultural revolution, the slow transition from hunting and gathering to crop growing and animal domestication, about 10000 BC to 8000 BC, the world population has been estimated at between 5 and 10 million; about 6000 BC, 200 million; about year 0 between 150 and 300 million; and about AD 1000 it was just over 300 million. Such early estimates vary greatly and are little more than informed guesses — but they provide rough indications. The rate of increase accelerated after AD 1000 and reached explosive proportions in quite recent times.

FIGURE 3: ESTIMATED WORLD POPULATION from AD 1000

FIGURE 4: ESTIMATED WORLD POPULATION GROWTH

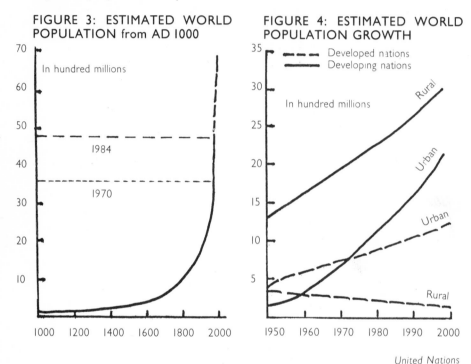

United Nations

This is shown in the population graphs (figures 3-6); the one of Great Britain, based on census returns, is the only one free of possible errors in estimation. In 1800, England was still a 'green and pleasant land', with a population of just under nine million; many of its rivers were abundant in salmon and its cities were still of human size; as Blake's often quoted lines remind us there were fields between Islington and 'Marybone', Primrose Hill and St John's Wood — though quite why he wanted to cover them with pillars of gold is not clear. The population is now about five times as large and many people live in cities of more than human size. It is a very much less pleasant land even if, for the time being, wealthier.

FIGURE 5: ESTIMATED WORLD POPULATION from 1650

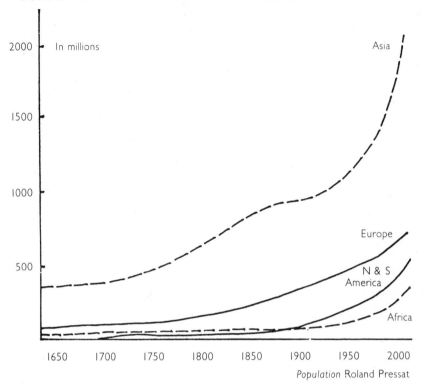

Population Roland Pressat

TABLE 3: WORLD POPULATION IN ROUND FIGURES

c. 1600 500 million
           Doubling period 230 years
1830 1000 million
           Doubling period 100 years
1930 2000 million
           Doubling period 46 years
1976 4000 million
           This represents an accelerating rate of exponential growth; normal exponential growth means a constant doubling period
1988 5000 million
2000 over 6000 million
           The last two figures are rough estimates or guesses based on a reduced annual rate of increase of just over 1.5% per year, as the **maximum** rate of increase was probably reached in about 1970

Britain with about two people per hectare is one of the most densely populated areas of the globe. The estimated world population in 1977 was 4,116 million, increasing then at about 1.5 million a week, 78 million a year or 1.9% per year (which means it would double every 37 years). The poorer countries are on the average increasing about twice as quickly as the richer ones. This book cannot look in detail at the reasons for population growth, but these include increasing life expectation and lower infant mortality. (SEE reading list).

FIGURE 6: POPULATION OF UNITED KINGDOM

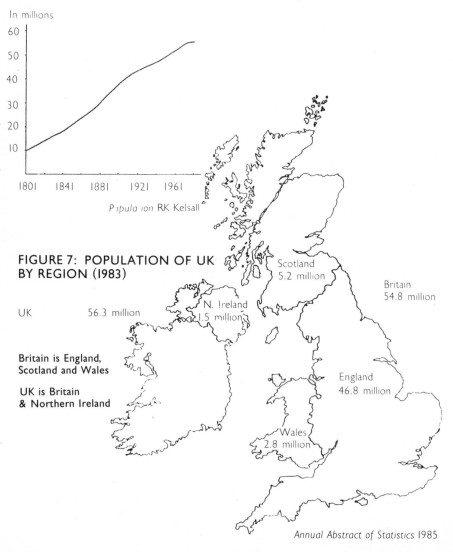

In millions

Popula ion RK Kelsall

FIGURE 7: POPULATION OF UK
BY REGION (1983)

UK   56.3 million

Britain is England,
Scotland and Wales

UK is Britain
& Northern Ireland

Scotland
5.2 million

Britain
54.8 million

N. Ireland
1.5 million

England
46.8 million

Wales
2.8 million

Annual Abstract of Statistics 1985

Urbanization

The population drift to the city is now world wide. There are now five cities in the world of more than 10 million (if urban agglomeration is included) and another six between 8 and 10 million; of the largest 15 cities only six are in the richer developed countries. The largest city in the world, when urban agglomeration is included, is New York. By the year 2000 it could well be Mexico City which has one of the fastest growing populations in the world and estimates indicate it could have 40 million by the turn of the century (*New Internationalist* no. 136, 1984).

TABLE 4: THE WORLD'S LARGEST CITIES

New York, USA	16.12 million
Mexico City, Mexico	14.75 million
Tokyo, Japan	11.68 million
Los Angeles, USA	11.49 million
Shanghai, China	10.82 million
Buenos Aires, Argentina	9.92 million
Calcutta, India	9.16 million
Paris, France	8.51 million
Seoul, South Korea	8.36 million
Moscow, USSR	8.39 million
Bombay, India	8.22 million
(London, United Kingdom	6.69 million)

UN Demographic Yearbook, 1982

Large cities are no utopias. Overcrowded human conditions produce their inevitable psychological reactions. For over 100 years now the drift has been from the country to the city and exploitation has probably as much or more to do with this than population increase. The megacity is a quite recent phenomenon, nineteenth century onwards; and may quite possibly be incapable of permanent survival. The population of ancient Rome at its height was probably less than a million and that of Constantinople in the seventh century less than half a million.

Demography and Malthus

John Gaunt's publication in 1662, based on weekly bulletins called 'Bills of Mortality' can be said to mark the start of demography. He was a prosperous London cloth merchant interested in social conditions and he studied these bulletins of births, deaths and causes of death, published by various London parishes, in a thoroughly scientific manner.

The name of Malthus, an English parson born in 1766, is much better known than that of Gaunt. His essay on the *Principlès of Population* published anonymously in 1798 ran into five editions by 1826. It was written as a reply to Godwin's *Enquiry Concerning Political Justice* (1793) and a similar French work by Candorcet — both were optimistic about the future and Godwin's outlook was equalitarian.

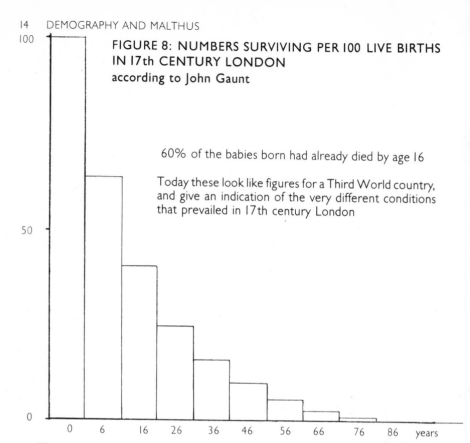

FIGURE 8: NUMBERS SURVIVING PER 100 LIVE BIRTHS
IN 17th CENTURY LONDON
according to John Gaunt

60% of the babies born had already died by age 16

Today these look like figures for a Third World country,
and give an indication of the very different conditions
that prevailed in 17th century London

The population of England had risen rapidly during the eighteenth century
(from about 5 million to 9.2 million) — the Enclosures had made matters
worse by reducing the overall food yield of the land, and the 'Poor Laws' which
entitled the poor to public assistance were becoming more costly to
taxpayers. (The cost rose from £2 million in 1785 to £4 million in 1801.)
Malthus wanted to abolish the Poor Laws. He argued that population
increases geometrically (and could double every 25 years) while food
production can only increase arithmetically and that therefore the inability to
produce enough food set an ultimate limit to the population.

He nevertheless opposed birth control and abortion and could shock
people then, as now, by statements more emotive than rational, like the
following:

'A man who was born into a world already possessed, if he cannot get
subsistence from his parents, on whom he has first demand, and if the
society do not want his labour, has no claim **of right** to the smallest
portion of food, and, in fact, has no business to be where he is. At
nature's mighty feast there is no vacant cover for him. She tells him to be
gone, and will quickly execute her own orders, if he does not work upon
the compassion of some of her guests'.

Without attempting a full conceptual analysis of this passage, it clearly assumes an almost divine right of property and employs the familiar propagandist's substitution trick — he introduces a personified divine 'Nature' to give false authority to his own crude opinions. It is an age old trick, still in constant use. It is not surprising that Malthus had many contemporary enemies and still has them. One wonders how, as a Church minister, he managed to reconcile his attitude with the teaching of Jesus and the communistic lifestyle of the early Church.

Malthus had also, no doubt, many friends among the rich, which was why his book sold so well. It provided a convenient false (moral?) excuse for the poverty of the many and the excessive wealth of a few (resulting from Enclosures and other forms of economic progress). Sixty years later Charles Darwin's *Origin of the Species* and the principle of 'natural selection' was to be used by 'philosophers' like Herbert Spencer to give a false pseudo-scientific excuse for the even greater excessive accumulations of wealth by a few due to industrialization, the development of America and so on, and the resulting impoverishment of the many. It was very popular among the 'robber baron' class in America (SEE for example, John K Galbraith *The Age of Uncertainty*).

Demography is now a much more sophisticated science. Simple models like that of Malthus are clearly inadequate. There can be, for example, great leaps forward as in the Green Revolution when in the developed world agricultural productive capacity more than doubled; while even expert short term population forecasts can be well out — one such in 1978, based on the Registrar General's figures, gave 60.8 million for the population of the UK in 1983; it was in fact 56.2 million. Still the rapid increase in the world population continues — the average annual growth rate of the world, still increasing, is nearly 2% and there are many signs of impending eco-catastrophe; for example the deserts are spreading in parts of Africa, due to destruction of trees for fuel, overgrazing of marginal land, and rapid population increase (4% per annum in some places).

THE ANIMAL POPULATION EXPLOSION AND ITS EXTRAVAGANT COST

The consequences of human population explosion are clear to all — they mean greater strain on the environment and the more rapid depletion of resources. The usual concomitant increase in numbers of animals reared for food greatly intensifies this, but tends to get taken for granted as many people still regard these animals as essential or desirable. But in fact such animals, bred and reared just for food, are both expensive and unnecessary. (Their numbers were very much less in Great Britain during the War when feeding people had priority over financial profit.) Collectively they eat much more plant food, about 5 to 10 times, than humans, and return as meat and dairy produce only a fraction of what they have eaten, probably on average no more than a tenth. Animal products need and use much more water than the equivalent vegetable food production. Where water supplies are scarce this involves more strain on water resources. Too many cattle destroy all grass and vegetation round a water hole in a very dry area and could result in permanent lowering of the water table. They are an unnecessary extravagance.

The animal centred diet has unfortunately acquired a prestige value and general acceptance, probably because it is very profitable — about two thirds of farmers' income comes from animal products, and others profit from their retail sale.

A meat and dairy diet requires much more land than a vegetarian or vegan diet would. (Vegans eat no animal produce whatever while vegetarians avoid meat and fish but eat eggs and dairy produce.) An American type diet requires 0.62 hectares per head, while a vegan diet would only need 0.08 hectares per head. There is **more than enough** arable land per head to support the world's human population, at the present level or at the foreseeable future level **on a vegan diet** but **nowhere near enough land for the extravagant animal produce centred** American one. The USA has a low population density (23 people per square kilometre), about one tenth of that of the UK, and a high agricultural productive capacity; it could afford something like its present style, but it still robs much poorer countries for extra meat or animal fodder, etc. So of course does the UK and other EEC countries. The EEC imports 60% of its oil seed and 90% of the proteins that British farmers, for example, turn extravagantly into very fatty foods. Britain imports some bread wheat but has no need to do so. The EEC is a large importer of agricultural products.

The price of the rich North's meat and animal produce centred diet (and wasteful lifestyle) is virtual murder. The best land in the Third World is used to grow cash crops for export, when it should be growing food for its own population. Their poorer farmers try to produce food on more marginal and arid land, but lack the resources to restore what they have taken out of it, even if this were always possible. Peasants have been driven also into the forests where the soil soon becomes exhausted. The Food and Agricultural Association (FAO) of the United Nations estimates that more than 111,370 square kilometres of forest world wide are being cleared each year to make way for agriculture. Every year 207,200 square kilometres (the area of England and Scotland combined) of previously fertile land declines to the state where it will yield nothing. (Alan Grainger Desertification Earthscan 1982)

DISTRIBUTION OF FOOD AND WEALTH

The Developed World and the Third World

Just over a quarter of the world's population of about 4.7 billion (1984) live in the richer north, while the poorer three quarters live (or exist) in the poorer south — in the area shaded on the map (Figure 9). In the richer developed world are the USA, Canada, the ten EEC countries, the USSR and associated East European states, other European countries, Japan, Australia, and New Zealand. Their average living standard is much higher than that of the Third World.

The United States with 5% of the world's population consumes nearly 40% of its resources (including all resources — not just food). It has a low population density and high agricultural potential output. It could easily feed many times its own population and imposes frequent restriction on agricultural production. On the other hand China feeds 22% of the world's population on only 7% of the world's cultivated area. (The large size of the country on the map is misleading as a large proportion of its total area, being mountainous or otherwise unsatisfactory, has little or no agricultural value.) It is trying to improve matters by using intensive methods to improve the soil, and the use of irrigation. It has had a rapidly increasing population, about 2.5% per year, and is taking strong measures to limit this growth.

FIGURE 9: THE RICH NORTH AND THE POOR SOUTH

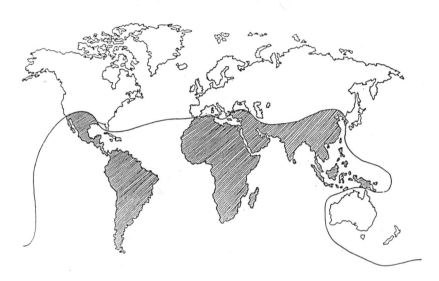

TABLE 5: THE RICH AND THE POOR

RICH PEOPLE | POOR PEOPLE

Gross national product per person (1981)
Richest 0.7 billion: $11,120 £7.943 p.a. | Poorest 2.2 billion: $270 £193 p.a.

Life expectation at birth (1981)
Richest 0.8 million: 74 years | Poorest 1.3 million: 47 years

Infant mortality: children dying before 1st birthday (1981)
Richest 0.8 million: 1% | Poorest 1.3 million: 14%

Percentage of available land (1983)
Richest 1.2 million: 43% | Poorest 3.5 million: 57%

Calorie intake per person (1980) as % of normal requirement
Richest 0.8 million: 133% | Poorest 1.3 million: 98.4%

New Internationalist June 1984

FIGURE 10: POPULATIONS OF THE RICH NORTH & THE POOR SOUTH

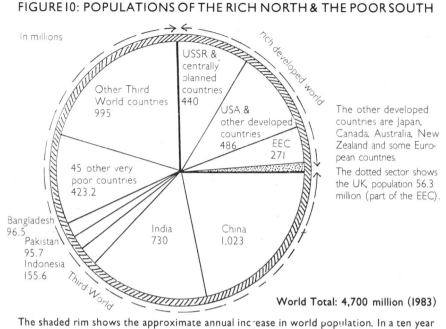

In millions

USSR & centrally planned countries 440

Other Third World countries 995

USA & other developed countries 486

EEC 271

45 other very poor countries 423.2

Bangladesh 96.5
Pakistan 95.7
Indonesia 155.6

India 730

China 1,023

The other developed countries are Japan, Canada, Australia, New Zealand and some European countries.

The dotted sector shows the UK, population 56.3 million (part of the EEC).

World Total: 4,700 million (1983)

The shaded rim shows the approximate annual increase in world population. In a ten year period it would be approximately 11 times thicker (compound interest rate of growth); in about 37 years the population, (represented by the area of the circle) would be doubled if the rate of increase remained constant (which is unlikely).

United Nations

Inequality between Individuals

The extreme inequality is not only between rich and poor nations — it is also between individuals in each. In Britain 95% of privately owned shares are owned by 5% of the population and this top 5% owns nearly half the personal wealth of the country. There is about the same inequality in the USA. In both countries the top 1% own about a quarter of the total wealth. One author in the British Association for the Advancement of Science book *Factory Farming* considers there could well be within the precincts of some oriental cities as many animals under cover as there were human beings sleeping in the open.

There are similar distributions of wealth in most 'free-enterprise' countries — though probably less unequal in 'planned economy' countries. There is an even greater inequality of wealth distribution in the poorer Third World countries and the consequences are much more dire there since the average level is so much lower. Thus though the calorie difference between the poorest and richest countries does not seem so extreme the protein supply difference will be much greater. Most citizens in the highly developed world get the recommended World Health Organization levels of protein and calories but only a minority of citizens of developing countries do.

The richest 20% of the world's population has 68% of the world income while the poorest 48% has 12% of the world income.

POPULATION AND POVERTY

The richest country in the world, the USA, has a high agricultural potential and only 25 people per square kilometre, while one of the poorest, Bangladesh (66% of whose land is arable) has 657 people per square kilometre (1983). Yet the Netherlands with 352 people per square kilometre is a prosperous land while Niger with only 5 per square kilometre is among the very poor countries of the world. However the latter country always had a low overall agricultural potential with low rainfall. In recent times, drought, over-grazing and cash crop production on the best land for export have made matters worse.

The large dairy production of the Netherlands is only possible because they import large quantities of animal feed. The claim of our Ministry of Agriculture (September 1985) for a high degree of self-sufficiency in indigenous type food — 81% (previous year 58%) — (although the trade deficit on non-indigenous type food has increased) is doubtful. We import bread wheat and fertilizer in large amounts. The claim also ignores the ecological damage of our intensive farming and the fantastic cost of farming subsidies. As far as self sufficiency is concerned it is worth noting that India has twice the available land per capita as China yet most visitors and experts agree that people in China no longer go hungry.

The density of the United Kingdom and India is similar (UK: 228 people per square kilometre; India: 223 people per square kilometre — 1983). In the eighteenth century there was probably little difference between the Gross National Product per capita of the UK and India; but now that of the UK is about 30 times as large. India has 15% of the world's population (732 million in 1983 — increasing at over 2% per year), 2.5% of its land area and a quarter of its cattle (the land of the 'sacred cow'). Until 1947 it was part of the British Empire; it is now a republic and member of the British Commonwealth. The population of the UK has been almost constant at near 56 million for about a decade.

The contrasts show that while population density is important there are other factors of equal importance, such as money to invest in improved methods of agriculture, foreign debts to be repaid out of production, and exploitation, both internal and external.

FIGURE II: POPULATION DENSITY AND WEALTH

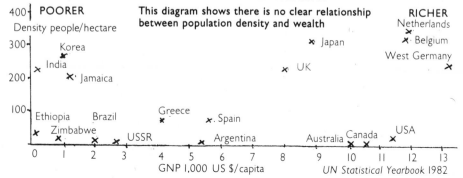

WHAT POPULATION COULD THE WORLD FEED?

The food the world already produces could feed all its present population, and more could easily be produced. The USA has more than once in recent decades cut back grain production. Could the Third World produce more? The answer is clearly that it could. Apart from land growing cash crops for export which could be used to grow food for local use, there is much unused cultivatable land in most of the poorer areas of the world. In the Introduction the case of people starving on or near first rate land was given which is a stark illustration of the exploitative misuse of land.

TABLE 6: CULTIVATED AND UNCULTIVATED LAND

	Australia & New Zealand	North America	South America	Europe	Africa	USSR	Asia	TOTAL
Total area million hectares	821	2108	1752	478	3019	2234	2736	
Area available for arable crops million hectares	154	465	680	174	732	356	627	3188
Area cultivated million hectares	16.2	239.8	76.9	153.8	157.8	226.6	518	1389
Proportion of land cultivated	11%	51%	11%	88%	22%	64%	83%	43.6%
Population 1982 millions	23.5	380	255	487	499	271	2672	4343.5
Cultivatable land /head hectares	6.54	1.25	2.59	0.36	1.47	1.31	0.23	0.73

Based on a table prepared for War on Want (1975) in Farming in the Clouds Richard Body

Studies carried out by the FAO and other agencies confirm there is much uncultivated land in the world. The World Food Problem: a report by the President's Science Advisory Committee showed that only about 44% of the world's potential arable land was actually being cultivated to grow crops.

Professor Roger Revelle in the Scientific American (September 1976) indicated that if all means of production were employed the world could feed 40 billion, even with some land still used for animal farming — 8 times its present population. On an entirely vegan diet it could feed still more. 'Food imports are in fact unnecessary. Our farm land is productive enough to support 250 million people on a vegetarian diet.' (British Medical Journal July 1977) The present population of the UK is 56 million (1985). Vegetarian here clearly means vegan.

Of course there is more to sustaining a population than just feeding: energy and resources are also involved and the present world population is if anything too high.

3 GROWTH, ECONOMICS AND NEOCOLONIALISM

RAPID GROWTH AND RESOURCES

There are two, often mentioned, models of the effects of rapid population increase. They have their uses and their limitations.

I THE EXPANDING LILY IN A POND OF LIMITED SIZE

A water lily in the centre of a pond, to start with, covers only one twentyfifth of its area (Fig. 12a). Suppose it doubles in size each month. After three months it still covers less than one third of the pond and after four months less than two thirds. But in the next 18 days it will fill the whole pond.

This is exponential growth, or growth at compound interest. It is what occurs initially when bacteria are grown in a culture, or approximately for the initial stage in the growth of a plant. Exponential decay (Fig. 12c) or decrease at a constant rate is important in the case of the decay of a radioactive substance or the cooling of a hot object. The growth of a tree or other plant will be as in figure 12d, it begins exponentially, slows down later and attains an almost constant final size.

FIGURE 12: EXPONENTIAL GROWTH

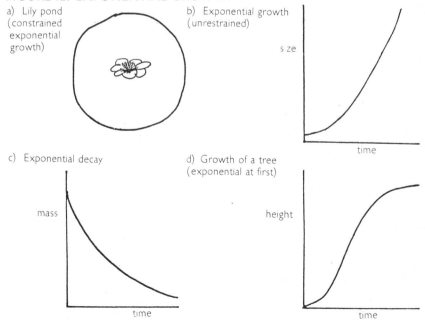

a) Lily pond (constrained exponential growth)

b) Exponential growth (unrestrained)

size

time

c) Exponential decay

mass

time

d) Growth of a tree (exponential at first)

height

time

When exponential or even more rapid rate of growth occurs it can cause an eco-catastrophe — like a plague of locusts. There is a natural penalty for being over-efficient parasites, whether paid for by the inevitable final rapid decline of insect pests or, for example, the pre-Revolution French kings and aristocracy.

The impossible results of sustained growth at compound interest (exponential growth) is illustrated by computing the value of £1 invested in the year 0 (1985 years ago) at 5% compound interest. It should now be worth £1.15 x 10^{42} which is about equivalent to a sphere of solid gold 1.75 times the diameter of the earth (or about 19 times its mass). If the initial £1 investment had been more recent, say in 1588 after the defeat of the Spanish Armada, it would in 1985 only amount to £258.3 million. Of course no investment in fact ever lasts a fraction of this time. There is inherent instability in any greed motivated economy.

Population for the world as a whole and for the separate continents and poorer countries has tended to resemble figure 12b but that of the UK and other developed countries is similar to figure 12d but the actual population graphs do not conform to any simple model. The lily pond model and figure 12d both have their limitations when applied to population increase.

II THE TRAGEDY OF THE COMMONS

This is another model of the inexorable result of growth producing overstrain and final destruction of resources. It was first outlined in 1833 by a mathematical amateur, William Foster Lloyd (1794-1852). A village community shares free and equal grazing rights on its common land. While the population remains small enough, and there are no over-greedy individuals, this causes few difficulties — and such a state could last for centuries (war and diseases can keep the numbers of humans down). But when the pressure on the land begins it will be more profitable for any individual to increase their own herd somewhat, even though this reduces the yield per unit of the whole; one individual gains, the loss is shared. This will clearly lead to overstrain on resources which could become catastrophic.

If the common lands were used in whole or part for vegetable growing the situation would be better. It provides no excuse whatever for the common land theft, euphemistically referred to as the 'Enclosures' (c. 1750-1850) which probably reduced areas of growing land and increased the grazing areas.

'The law does punish man or woman,
Who steals the goose from off the Common
But lets the greater felon loose,
Who steals the Common from the goose.'

The tragedy of the commons paradigm applies to such shibboleth notions as 'the freedom of the seas' and 'inexhaustible resources of the sea' which have brought the whale and species after species of fish near to extinction, and to the horror of the periodical seal 'culls'. It applies even to such matters as traffic congestion in city centres; each individual can go more quickly in their own car than by bus, but as a result lengthens the time of the journey for all whether by bus or by car.

The inexorable nature of the tragedy of the commons as far as grazing is concerned depends on the assumption that we need so many, or even any, domestic food animals.

ECOLOGY AND CONVENTIONAL ECONOMICS

Ecology is a term taken over from biology where it referred to the dynamic equilibrium of plants, animals and other living organisms, in their natural habitat. In the last few decades the term has acquired a much extended meaning and has come to centre on the effects of the most greedy and destructive animal in nature on the local and global environment. A term which implied a detached objective study of flora and fauna in their natural surroundings and the ecocycles into which they fit, was even applied to a political party — the 'Ecology Party' in Britain, now the 'Green Party'.

Social and political ecology could be described as sane economics in contrast to the money centred or mammon worship of the conventional economists; for money and the profit motive distort and destroy real values. Conventional economics makes much of sustained economic growth, booms, recessons, depressions, interest rates, rates of exchange, rates of inflation, etc. in terms which suggest that such notions are inescapable natural phemonena, instead of the results of ill-contrived, ill-inspired human devices.

We live in a world of introverted values; people are referred to by the degrading term consumers (like silk worms consuming mulberry leaves), bits of an economic machine designed to 'create wealth' (meaning 'make money for me and my friends'). The whole attitude of politicians, mass media and opinion engineers generally is that industries, including agriculture, exists to make profits and employ people instead of to provide food, houses, clothing etc. and services for people. This wrong attitude is universal, it runs through the publications of the NEDO (National Economic Development Office) and other official publications and is implicit in the speeches of politicians, CBI (Confederation of British Industry) spokesmen, union leaders, etc. Policies based on false values are not likely to produce results.

Meanwhile on a global ecological scale, there is the gradual spread of deserts in Africa and elsewhere, the use of the best land in hungry countries to produce cash crops for export, the heavy debts of poorer countries, so that a large proportion of their hard produced exports are used merely to keep pace with interest charges, and above all the continual destruction of the world's 'lungs' and world weather regulator, the tropical rain forests.

The *New Internationalist* (December 1982) in an article dealing with population pressure on already meagre land holdings quotes a young woman in Kenya:

'My life is very different from my mother's. Life is much more difficult now because everyone is dependent on money. Long ago money was unheard of. No one needed it. But now you can't even get food without cash. Times are very difficult.'

Improved health care here has caused population growth, less land per head, hence less food and real income. This has increased the importance of wages and cash and raised the status of the wage earner. (There is also the factor of soil deterioration. Kenya like other parts of Africa has problems of drought resulting from wholesale tree destruction — a subject to be considered later.)

That people could manage even in the 20th Century without any money makes a nonsense of the kind of 'economic' arguments to which we are treated daily by the mass media.

THE RISKS OF CONVENTIONAL POLICIES

There is a great moral gap between the world of the old individualistic values of conventional economics and those of the social ecological outlook; a difference recognised by forward looking people, including some prominent politicians, as the fairly conservative Brandt report showed. The danger of eventual Third World reaction has been seen for some time. U Thant, Secretary General of the United Nations from 1961 to 1971, warned of the dangers of leaving effective action on Third World injustice too long. Giscard d'Estaing suggested the possibility of the Third World later on taking revenge on the highly developed world for 19th century exploitation and its present attitude. One could add — for its present money-lending exploitation. In fact a contemporary focus of attention (1984) is the matter of the indebtedness of the poorer countries to the overwealthy 'North'.

This links in with the issues of cash crops, the ecological damage to soil etc. due to poverty in the Third World, the ever growing menace of the new super powers, the transnationals (or multinationals) and the spread of nuclear weapons and other sophisticated armaments everywhere.

Third World countries or rather their governments (generally composed of their rich minorities — or worse) are persuaded to purchase expensive military hardware when the scarce resources so used should have been employed to provide adequate food, better health and education services, adequate housing and clean water supplies.

'In recent years over 100 British Aerospace Hawk ground attack aircraft have been sold to Third World countries by Britain. For the cost of one of these Hawks, one and a half million people could be provided with clean safe water.'

Campaign against the Arms Trade

And Britain is only one of the 'merchants of death'. 80% of UK arms exports go to Third World countries; and other rich overdeveloped countries are also involved in this trade.

'In 1982 when other tensions were perhaps more dangerous than East-West conflict $650 billion were spent world wide on military purposes, adding to an arsenal already capable of destroying human kind many times over.'

Common Crisis: the second Brandt report

President Reagan has subsidized the nuclear industry in the USA to an extent where they can almost afford to give away a reactor to a Third World country and actively seek Third World markets. Only five countries (USA, USSR, China, France and Great Britain) have atomic weapons, but those who have the capability to produce them include Israel, South Africa, Pakistan, India, Argentina, Brazil, South Korea and Taiwan — with many more probables. Since any nuclear reactor, even a research reactor, can be used to produce material for nuclear weapons the number of states possessing nuclear weapons will increase.

NEOCOLONIALISM AND ECOLOGICAL ERRORS

Neocolonialism, the use of economic pressure by powerful countries to dominate much poorer developing ones, has now largely replaced the previous military dominance; (except in Central and South America where the USA employs both forms of persuasion — as does also the other contemporary large imperialist power, the USSR, in Afghanistan and elsewhere. Both empires have been gradually expanding during the last two centuries).

FOOD POWER

The main staple grain exporting countries of the world are the USA, Canada, Australia and Argentina. They can use their food surplus as an instrument of considerable power (though massive debts reduce Argentina's influence). Earl Butz, US Secretary of State for Agriculture in 1974 said 'Food is a weapon, it is now one of the principal weapons in our negotiating kit'. This was in reply to the OPEC (Organization of Petroleum Exporting Countries) countries mutual agreement on oil prices (or 'cornering the oil market' — according to point of view). In November 1974, US Assistant Secretary of State, Thomas O. Enders, spoke of the food producers' monopoly exceeding the oil producers' and stressed its power to influence, and President Ford (September 1974) at the United Nations spoke in similar terms.

In 1980, after the Russian invasion of Afghanistan, the USA put an embargo on all sales of grain to the USSR not already pledged by contract. It was not very effective and would have had no effect whatever if Russia did not consume excessive amounts of meat and animal products. It would have had a devastating effect on a poor developing country and none would therefore act so as to provoke such an embargo.

In fact poor Third World countries find it difficult to pay for necessary food imports but in recent years have been driven to do so, paid for by aid or loans. Such imports are only 'necessary' because of mismanagement and exploitation both internal and external. Thus as the second Brandt report (*Common Crisis*) points out, African countries are now on average importing 8% to 9% of their food — even though two thirds of their labour force is engaged in agriculture. The rich countries dominate the markets in which poor countries must compete, and since the poor countries start so far behind, and many have high population growth, they may find it impossible to catch up. This means that price levels will be set by the purchasing power of the rich countries with disastrous results.

> 'In 1960 three tons of bananas were enough to buy a tractor . . . in 1970 it needed eleven tons for a tractor. This is the position with most Third World exports and their manufactured imports.'
>
> War on Want *Outlook* no. 4
>
> 'In 1960, 8.3 tonnes of rubber could earn enough to buy two tractors. In 1975 two tractors cost as much as 25 tonnes of rubber.'
>
> *Oxfam Atlas*

According to *Common Crisis* between June 1980 and June 1982 the price of sugar (outside special arrangements) fell 78%, rubber by 37% and copper by 35%. This makes the struggle even more difficult for Third World countries. Subsidized exports by rich developed countries hurt poor developing countries' exports to world markets. Subsidized EEC sugar exports rose to 18.3% of the world market in 1981. And this is only part of the injust treatment of the Third World by the rich countries. In fact to call it 'injust' is an understatement. Very many sugar producers in poor countries will have been ruined by this diabolical nonsense, and many workers made destitute. It will also have cost EEC taxpayers and consumers large sums of money. (If there is one 'food' in which self sufficiency has no value it is sugar.)

Statistics for food exports and imports are misleading. Almost the whole of North, Central and South America has a surplus in food exports; so has much of Africa, India, Indonesia and the Phillipines and Australia and New Zealand. But many of these countries (apart of course from USA, Canada, Australia and New Zealand) are very poor and contain many under-nourished people. The overall surplus is often due to large exports of single crops, like coffee, tea, cocoa, sugar, honey or tropical fruits — cash crops in fact. Those with a food export deficit (food importers) on the other hand include many of the richer countries of the world; Europe, USSR, OPEC countries, Japan and China (China being the exception here). Other apparent exceptions in Europe — Ireland, Netherlands and Denmark — are so in money terms only; they really import both more protein and more energy (calories), in the form of grain and animal fodder, than they produce in the form of meat and dairy produce, but the latter has a higher market value. A reasonably equable and prosperous society ensures that the profits from these virtual 'cash crops' are spread among the community.

The example of Guinea Bissau highlights many of the worst features of neocolonialism. It was recently brought to light by Wyndham James, Oxfam's former West African Field Director. Balance of payments difficulties, due to falling commodity prices, persuaded the government of Guinea Bissau to ban all sale of peanuts locally, although at certain times they could form a crucial source of protein, especially for children. So they are exported; most come to

Europe and feed our pigs and our cows, and so help to produce the Common Market milk surplus; they may then return as dried milk for malnourished children with a small fraction of their total nutritional value and with a false label of 'charitable' aid.

This example exposes the root cause of the hunger problem: POVERTY. The rich 'North' exploit the poor 'South' countries while the rich in each country exploit their own poor. Much of the best land in many Third World countries and land where average rainfall is generally adequate is given over to cash crops. And this is so because the land is owned by a minority of rich people who put profit before the nutritional welfare of poor people. A result of bad government and neocolonialism.

CASH CROPS

Crops like tea, coffee, sugar, cotton, cocoa, in the Third World take up land that could grow food. Such crops are of course more valuable in cash terms than the food; but the profit does not go to the Third World country but to the rich world based multinationals who usually pay very low wages to their workers. In 1984 Zimbabwe had to import 400,000 tonnes of maize but had record crops of tobacco, cotton and soya beans for export. Kenya in the same year suffered from drought but as an Oxfam consultant pointed out the areas of best rainfall grew cash crops for export including luxury items like strawberries and asparagus.

During the last twenty years Africa has doubled sugar cane output and quadrupled tea production. Non-food crops occupy over 25% of the area in the Third World used for crop production (mainly for export). The area used for soya bean cultivation in India (mostly for export) increased five times from 1974 to 1982. In the Philippines (a very poor country) one third of all cultivated land is used to grow food for export while many of its own inhabitants are not adequately fed.

In addition the prices of most of the developing world's outputs have tended to decline relative to their imports. Third World producers of bananas, cotton, jute, rubber and tea have seen the purchasing power of their exports decline steadily in the last twenty years.

The fact however remains that dire poverty, debt repayments, extremely uneven distribution of purchasing power and the insatiable greed of rich countries cause poor countries to produce cash crops on land which could grow food for their own people. It is also a fact that these same conditions cause overuse of marginal lands and clearing of forest. In semi-arid zones, which form about a fifth of the earth's surface, overfarming, overgrazing, overpopulation and deforestation can produce desert.

Tea

Tea is a cash crop of special interest as the United Kingdom is still easily the world's largest importer (149,000 tonnes in 1978, but declining annually). India is both the largest consumer and producer. The tea trade is an example of ruthless exploitation with very large profits and extremely low wages, bad housing for workers and neglect of workers' health; all of course in very poor countries with high rates of unemployment (it is at least 40% in Sri Lanka). *The Tea Trade* is a well researched, concise booklet by the World Development Movement (WDM). It deserves to be widely read. In 1979 WDM members, who had purchased shares for this purpose, attended the Annual General Meeting of James Finlay in Glasgow and accused the firm of paying tea pickers in Bangladesh only 20p a day; this produced the required press publicity and adverse comment. The comments of Finlay chairman, Sir Colin Campbell, did little to counter balance the adverse publicity; 'nobody is forced to work for us' he said, 'we go to seek a fortune for our stockholders in many parts of the world and when in Rome do as the Romans do'. Sir Colin, known as 'Sir Cumference' in Kenya because of his bulk, was being paid £23,000 a year.

In spite of the huge profits involved and the appalling wages, housing and shameful neglect of the health of the tea pickers it is not the worst of the cash crops. More than 50% of the price of a tea packet finds its way back to its producing country compared with about 10% of the cost of a bunch of bananas. All the same, about 25% of the price of a quarter of tea goes to pay for blending and packaging in Britain. The WDM through Traidcraft and TradeFair sell tea packed in Sri Lanka thus increasing the benefit to the people there. (Addresses at the back of this book.) They also sell other goods produced in the Third World.

'Cotton or Food for Tanzania'

A story which illustrates the ecological consequences of intensive exploitation of the land for financial gain in the form of the cash crop, cotton, is given in an article by Paula Park in *Oxfam News*, winter 1984.

Sade Jima moved in the fifties as a small child with her father from Singida to Shinyanga in central Tanzania. The land in Singida 'was so dry that we could only grow groundnuts. We heard that in Shinyanga people were raising cotton and making lots of money. At the time, when the first rains came in November, all the trees blossomed and grass began to grow. We ploughed the ground and in a month's time, planted. We harvested maize, millet, mangoes and bananas — food of all kinds — in addition to cotton. Now no one knows when the rain will fall, or how long it will last. We plant food at the first rains, but often the seeds die and we have to replant; sometimes we harvest nothing'.

Her region is one that will receive emergency food this year. There has been next to no food harvest but it has been a bumper year for cotton. Tanzania has developed drought resistant strains of millet, sorghum and cotton, but cotton is the most effective. Cotton takes much from the soil but is still the priority for the Ministry of Agriculture. Trees have disappeared due to intensive cultivation and the stripping of land by fire. Sade's problem today is growing food. In her words 'there were trees by the riverside which seems to attract the rain because that area was always the wettest. Now the trees are gone'.

Long term ecological considerations have been sacrificed to short term financial gains; and the interests of rural areas to those of urban.

The Bangladesh Frog Massacre

Ag Scene (newsletter of 'Compassion in World Farming) (July 1984) gives an account of the frog massacre in India and Bangladesh. Damp low lying areas in these countries support a large population of large hungry frogs which are among the peasant farmers' best friends. They eat close on their own body weight of insects and other crop pests each day as well as the carriers of cattle-afflicting water-borne diseases and insects that carry malaria and encephalitis. It is an ecological crime of the first order to attack them but they are being ruthlessly and cruelly slaughtered to provide 'delicacies' for 'gourmets' in France and Britain. (The French have eaten their own supplies to near extinction and the few survivors there are protected by legislation.) The cruelty of this slaughter is revolting. Live and conscious frogs are cut in two by pushing them against a fixed vertical blade; the top half which survives for minutes is just discarded and the legs only are used. India exported 3,570 tonnes in 1978, which is the equivalent of 10,700 tonnes of live frogs which could have eaten 10,000 tonnes of crop pests per day had they been alive in the rice paddies and coconut gardens.

Even in simple monetary terms this trade is a dead loss, because the £5.5 million in foreign exchange obtained from the frogs' legs export is offset by a £13 million bill for imported pesticides, to do the work the dead frogs would have done for nothing, according to Dr. A. Joshi of Bombay Natural History Society — and some of these pesticides are so dangerous that they have been banned from the West. No doubt the political voice of the frogs' legs exporters is louder than that of the peasants who will have to pay the cost of the pesticides — the Indian Prime Minister, Desai, would like a ban on this export, but is apparently unable to introduce one due to political pressures. However, in India, frogs are to be stunned prior to slaughter.

It is a remarkable comment on the misuse of aid to note that in 1983 the EEC aid programme funded a trade mission for Bangladesh exporters of frozen frogs' legs to visit Britain, France, Germany and Italy to find new buyers.

Meat

Meat is also a cash crop with the usual properties thereof — it is an expensive 'luxury' item, which uses land of the poorer country (which could be better employed); it is exported to a richer one, which does not **need** it, while so-called market forces ensure the poorer country gets the minimum price for its produce. The export of beef cattle from Costa Rica, Guatemala, Honduras and Nicaragua increased five times between 1960 and 1980 to 110,000 tonnes a year. (Since the 1979 revolution in Nicaragua cattle exports have declined greatly and food production has increased.) These cattle are grass fed and so leaner than the mainly grain fed animals of the USA to where they mostly go; they are also much cheaper and like other Third World exports keep declining in cash value. (The money value of a tonne of beef export in 1981 from a Third World country was about 11% of its value in 1971.) This fact, together with the 'debt trap' in which so much of the Third World finds itself, means these beef exports continue to expand, resulting in less land for home produced food crops for home consumption, and this is the position regarding other cash crops.

> Cash crops are subsidies from a number of poor countries given to rich consuming nations. When peanuts or soya (good sources of protein for humans) are imported from poor countries to feed cattle to produce, as in the EEC, surplus milk and butter it is just crazy economics.

Cash crops like cotton, tea and tobacco give higher yields in tropical countries but use up soil nutrients more rapidly than most food crops. They therefore need regular additions of fertilizer if the soil is not to become exhausted, which adds to the capital outlay of growing them. Pesticides, usually also required, add more to the outlay cost. Large quantities of pesticides are used throughout the 7 or 8 months growing period of tobacco — often carelessly; the World Health Organization estimates that one person in the developing world is poisoned by pesticides every minute of every day. Cotton covers 5% of the world's cultivated land area, and uses more pesticide than any other crop. The capital intensive system, using expensive hybrid seeds, fertilizers and pesticides, but less labour, leads to larger and larger farms. Numerous small peasant farmers who could generally produce all their own food, and more, have been displaced, and their land and wealth accumulate in the hands of a few. In north east Brazil, for example, 9% of land owners now possess nearly 82% of the land and just 15 landowners occupy almost as much land as the total owned by the 363,776 small holders. The inequality in land distribution is as bad in the UK (SEE Land distribution and use) but as few here depend directly on the land and there is a welfare state it has less dire results.

Producing cash crops frequently ensures the grower an instant, profitable market, via wealthy transnational organizations, while disposing of a food crop locally may take time — an important consideration to a grower working on restricted credit. Transnationals are often, of course, land owners and growers, so that a previous colony may by this means virtually remain one.

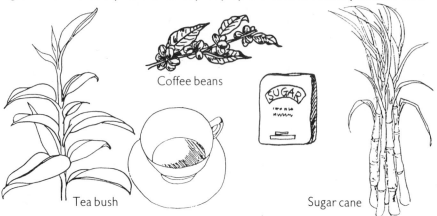

Coffee beans

Tea bush   Sugar cane

EXPLOITATION IN BRAZIL

Brazil is another example of neocolonial exploitation, of the dire need of some due to others' greed. Drought in the north east of the country has recently (1984) focussed world attention, but this is by no means the whole story which Oxfam describes as an 'Unnatural Disaster'. Brazil (8.5 million square kilometres) is the largest country in South America (17.8 million sq. km.) with just under half its area, and just under half its population (115 million out of 236 million in 1978). It has a high rate of population increase — 2.8% per annum, which means it would double in 25 years. It is potentially a most prosperous country, rich in natural resources and a high agricultural output; but is has also the world's largest debt burden of £80 billion (end of 1983). It is one of the largest food exporting countries and has at the same time very high and extensive rates of malnutrition. An Oxfam survey in Ceara State in the North East showed half the children were malnourished. Some areas report 25% infant mortality rates. People in the North East have a life expectancy of only 50 years, but malnutrition is not only in the drought stricken areas. (Source: *Unnatural Disaster* Oxfam) Brazil also has the widest income disparity of any country in the world: the wealthiest 20% of the population has an average income 33 times that of the poorest 20% (1984). In the United Kingdom the corresponding figure is 6 and in the USA, 11.

Brazil has a large trade export surplus; recent trade surpluses are about double previous years, but will be used up by interest repayments on debts — about £12 billion. Some 40 million people live in conditions of extreme poverty, nearly 75% of the population is getting rapidly poorer, the rate of inflation was about 200% in 1983 (official rate 150%). In 1983 beans went up 769% and rice went up 188%. Various studies have shown that large numbers — up to two thirds — of the population are not eating sufficient to satisfy the World Health Organization's recommended calorie intake. Desperate situations provoke desperate responses; in the North East raids on supermarkets, small shops and food stores have increased. There were 43 such raids in the state of Pernambuco in 1983; in the first two months of 1984 there were 42.

AGRIBUSINESS, BIG MONEY AND MULTINATIONALS

Agribusiness is **big** business in the products of agriculture. On a world scale it is mainly in the hands of a small number of large multinationals. In 1971 the annual production of the world's top ten multinationals was greater than the gross national product of each of 80 sovereign states. The worst effects of their operations are felt far more in the poor nations than in the rich world. Any rich world mongrel or pampered puss today is a better customer for agribusiness than a poor human being. In 1807 Hazlitt replying to Parson Malthus states that 'the dogs and horses of the rich eat up the food of the children of the poor', so the situation is by no means new, but today it is on a much larger scale.

The ever-increasing power of the multinationals or transnationals, and the great money assets of the big banks and the crushing burden of their loans to the Third World, are frightening in their potential consequences. In 1977, there were 15 transnationals in the USA, 14 in Europe, in Japan, Venezuela and Iran one each, with annual sales income over $8 billion. The largest, Exxon, USA based, had an annual sales income of $44.8 billion. Although transnationals operate world-wide, the home bases of the world's largest (over $1 billion per year sales income) are in the USA (about 60%), West Europe (including UK) (about 30%) and Japan (about 10%).

In 1977 the sales income of Mobil ($26.06 billion) and the other top ten transnationals exceeded the gross national product (GNP) of all African states except South Africa. GNP is by no means a perfect measure of the total wealth of a country but it does give a rough indication thereof, and the comparison with the sales income of the transnationals does highlight their fantastic power. By 1980, the world's top 30 transnationals had more than 25,000 affiliates with combined sales of $2,700 billion, six times Britain's national income. The comparison between bank assets and national resources is an even rougher indication but again it shows their enormous power. In 1976 no state in the world had reserves greater than the assets of the Bank of America (then the world's largest bank) $73,913 million, and only West Germany had reserves greater than the assets of the National Westminster Bank (then the 20th), $29,0800 million, while many states in South America and Africa had resources below the assets of the Cantonal Bank of St Gall (then the 300th in size) $1,707 million. (Sources: *State of the World Atlas*, Government Statistical Service).

FIGURE 13: BIG COMPANIES, SMALL COUNTRIES

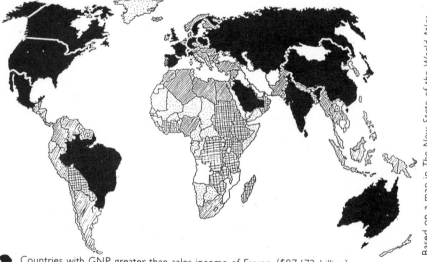

Based on a map in *The New State of the World Atlas*

⬛ Countries with GNP greater than sales income of Exxon ($97.172 billion)

▨ GNP above sales income of ICI ($12.873 billion) but less than that of Exxon

▦ GNP above sales income of Philippine National Oil ($2.890 billion) but below that of ICI

⋮⋮ GNP less than sales income of Philippine National Oil ☐ GNP not available for comparison

About one fifth of consumer spending in the UK goes on food, although agricultural production is only about 3% of the GNP. Rank-Hovis-McDougall, Associated British Foods and Spillers French have about 75% of the British market for bread or flour; for margarine Unilever have 70% and Nestles 20%; for sugar Tate and Lyle have 60% and many other foods are also dominated by a few large firms.

World wide the powerful multinationals have a monopoly, or near monopoly, of many foods — many multinationals are also in other lines of business. Unilever, the ninth largest multinational (worldwide) is the first in agribusiness. Its base is in Western Europe but it operates in 15 European countries, 16 countries in North and South America, 29 countries in Africa, 12 in Asia and 2 in Australasia. It is truly international. It claims 500 subsidiaries but records at Companies House, London, showed Unilever Ltd., London, has 812 subsidiaries and there are other subsidiaries of Unilever N.V. Rotterdam. Its main turnover is in food, followed by detergents and toiletries, paper, plastics and packing, plantations abroad and animal feeds. Counter Information Services have a 102 page booklet on Unilever (with a three page list of some of its subsidiaries). They also have information on other multinationals.

COMMERCIOGENIC MALNUTRITION

This is a name coined for the type of undernourishment produced or generated by commercial forces and the pressure of the 'ad men'. When people in Bangladesh are persuaded (by advertisers) to buy processed baby food when they could buy cow's milk much cheaper, or breast-feed, we have an example of the effects of disturbing established habits for commercial gain. Disturbing an established unsophisticated food pattern is often disastrous. Tooth decay has grown rapidly over the last two centuries – probably due to increased use of white sugar and white flour and highly refined food. Fluoride is no answer to this problem. However in Britain tooth decay is now declining. HMS *Carlisle* called at the island of Tristan da Cunha in 1932 — the ship's surgeon examined the teeth of the 162 inhabitants; 83% were entirely free from defect, no child under 5 had bad teeth. When the *Carlisle* called again in 1937 no less than 50% of the population had one or more bad teeth. Several ships had called in the meantime bringing in white sugar and white flour. Similar results came from the French occupation of Tahiti — French cuisine had a disastrous effect on the hitherto perfect teeth of the natives.

The worst ideas from the industrialized world sometimes spread most rapidly in the Third World and factory farming is certainly one of them. Battery poultry production units from Japan to Bangladesh in 1979 is a recent example of a most undesirable export from a rich to a very poor country. The spread of the harmful smoking habit in the Third World is another. A Mexican rural sociologist found that the two products which peasants want to buy the moment they come in contact with the advertising message are white bread and soft drinks — two of our most undesirable products nutritionally in a poor country.

Commerciogenic malnutrition is a most malevolent export of the rich world to the Third World. Persuading their less sophisticated citizens, by advertising pressure, that their traditional foods are somehow inferior, can undermine their health. Doctors working in rural Mexican villages report that a family may often sell its few eggs and chickens to buy Coke for the father while the children waste away for lack of protein. Other cases are given in Susan George's book *How the Other Half Dies*.

The Baby Food Scandal

In 1973 the *New Internationalist* published the first accounts of the Nestles baby food scandal. Malnutrition in the developing world had been greatly added to by the increased misuse of artificial feeding; babies in some African hospitals were in beds marked 'Lactogen Syndrome' after the Nestles baby food of that name. Nestles is the world's second largest agribusiness. *The Baby Killer*, published by War on Want in 1974, dealt with the bad effects of powdered milk in the Third World, but the scandal continued as *The Baby Killer Scandal* (1979) showed. The situation in 1985 is better than it was then . . . as a result of sustained pressure.

The International Baby Foods Action Network (IBFAN) was set up by a range of non-Governmental organisations and other interested parties to lobby the European Parliament and so get through measures to control the sale and use of powdered milk. The Code of Marketing of Breast Milk Substitutes (set up in 1981) involves the encouraging of breast feeding, and of weaning practices suitable to available local food resources, the improved health of women, and the marketing and distribution of infant formulae and weaning goods.

In February 1984 Nestles agreed to conform to the International Code of Marketing and the International Baby Milk Action Coalition suspended its six month's boycott. The Code of Marketing is still mainly voluntary but Nestles is now one of the more co-operative of the multinationals. Only 12 countries have formally adopted the Code and fewer still have made it legally binding. Britain has adopted a watered down version after representations made by British baby milk companies.

While the situation is better than it was, an unpublished study by IBFAN reveals there were over 500 breaches of the WHO baby milk marketing code in 12 Third World countries in just two months of 1984 (Source: John Tanner *Spur* WDM, Dec 84/Jan 85)

4 THE POLITICAL BACKGROUND

THE MAKING OF WORLD POVERTY

There is a consensus of opinion in the developed affluent world that assumes the Third World has always been poor and that development comes from the 'North' to save the 'South'. The Brandt Commission report (SEE later) carefully avoids the historic reasons for contemporary poverty and the consequences of past colonialism and present neocolonialism. Thus for example, the Brandt Report says 'focussing on questions of historical guilt will not provide answers to the crucial problem of self-responsibility on which alone mutural respect can build. Self-righteousness will neither create jobs nor feed hungry mouths'. This is entirely 'Eurocentric' in outlook. The 'historical guilt' means the record of Britain and other colonizing nations in impoverishing the Third World, and so creating its present poverty. The rest of the first sentence quoted, in its context, means the Third World should emulate the progressive developed world and profit by 'mutual' trade. The 'mutual' advantage of north–south trade is a central theme of the Report though in fact north–south trade is to the invariable financial advantage of the 'North'.

Facts of historical guilt and European colonial exploitation founded on violence do provide most of the explanation for the present tragic state of the world. Of course the self-righteous myopia of the previous exploiting groups will avoid seeing this. A century or so ago in empire building days, moral myopia had an arrogant rather than a self-justifying guise. Cecil Rhodes in 1896 described the Empire as somewhere to settle our surplus population and as a market for goods produced in our factories and mines. 'If there be a God, I think what he would like me to do is to paint as much of the map of Africa British red as possible'. The inferior countries were to be a convenience for the superior British people.

The scope of this book does not permit a full or adequate account of colonial exploitation. *The Creation of World Poverty* by Teresa Hayter gives an excellent and concise account of this, and much of this section is drawn from this book, which shows how Britain and other colonizing powers have damaged and destroyed industries in the countries they ruthlessly exploited — how for example the British destroyed the cotton trade of India.

Between 1815 and 1832 the value of Indian cotton goods exported fell from £1.3 million to below £100,000; the value of English cotton goods imported by India rose from £156,000 in 1794 to £400,000 in 1832. By the mid nineteenth century India was importing a quarter of all British cotton exports. Even in India taxes effectively discriminated against local cloth. The East India Company protested against this — their trading profits were decreased. Sir Charles Trevelyan declared to a parliamentary enquiry in 1840, 'the population of Dacca has fallen from 150,000 to 30,000 or 40,000 and the jungle and malaria are fast encroaching upon the town . . . Dacca which used to be the Manchester of India has fallen off from a flourishing town to a poor and small one'. 'The bones of the weavers are bleaching the plains of India' wrote a Governor General of the East India Company in 1836. The Indian iron and steel industry was destroyed like the textile one — by the use of selective duties in each direction.

It is absurd to pretend this is irrelevant to the present state of India or that the Spanish conquests in Central and South America are to the present unhappy state of these countries. The Spaniards in the Americas are estimated to have killed 12 to 15 million; densely populated areas like Haiti, Cuba, Nicaragua and the coast of Venezuela were completely depopulated. Europeans with their conceit and ruthless arrogance and their self-protective myopic deception, destroyed the indigenous cultures and economies of four continents. For every dollar US companies invest in Latin America three dollars come back in profit. Nathaniel Davies, US ambassador in Guatemala, said in the US Chamber of Commerce in 1971, 'Money isn't everything, love is the other two per cent. I think that characterizes the United States' relationship with Latin America'.

WHAT IS THE 'GROUP OF 77'?

This is an association of developing nations — the original 77 has expanded to 126 (1983) — from Brazil to the tiny state of Vanuatu, formed to seek a better deal for the world's poorer nations and realizing that unity is strength. They aim to shake up the powerful rich nations as the trade unions have shaken up the entrepreneur classes within the industrialised nations. They have the support of OPEC and some of their members are exporters of metals and other materials vital to the rich world's industrial production and economies. Some also are increasing their own industrial production.

THE INTERNATIONAL MONETARY FUND (IMF) AND THE WORLD BANK (IBRD)

These were both set up by the United Nations Monetary and Financial Conference of 44 nations which met at Bretton Woods, New Hampshire, USA in July 1944. Both began to function in December 1945. They are both specialized agencies of the UN but also independent organizations. IBRD stands for International Bank for Reconstruction and Development. The International Development Association (IDA) (which began operating in November 1960) and the International Finance Corporation (IFC, July 1956) are regarded as parts of the World Bank. The IDA lends at nominal interest rates to the poorest countries. Its loans are about 31% of World Bank lending. The IFC assists private investment in Third World lending (about 6%). The IDA is aid funded; the IBRD and IFC are not. The World Bank funded the Kariba Dam, the Volta Dam (Ghana) and large power plants in India, Pakistan and Latin America. At present it provides about half of all international aid for agriculture in the Third World.

In its early years the IMF sorted out balance of payments deficits in Europe in a then world of fixed exchange rates, acting as a bank lending interim loans. Its operations today are world wide but most voting power is vested in the twenty rich industrial countries involved (58%) (SEE figure 14) It has lent billions of dollars to Third World countries, and imposed harsh economic policy measures therewith. In the last six years there has been rioting in Peru, Turkey, Jamaica and now Brazil as a result.

FIGURE 14: IMF COMPOSITION AND VOTING POWER

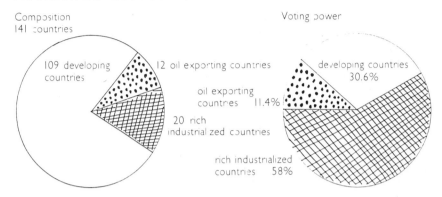

Composition
141 countries

109 developing countries

12 oil exporting countries

20 rich industrialized countries

Voting power

developing countries 30.6%

oil exporting countries 11.4%

rich industrialized countries 58%

While there are all the same many poor countries applying for loans, the Sandinistas in Nicaragua determined to have nothing to do with the IMF and were doubtful about the World Bank. When a Filippino revolutionary was asked whether the left should try to borrow from the Bank when it won power he said he would prefer 'not to ride the tiger'.

There is a difference of view here but perhaps less than at first sight. Aid should be given without strings attached and should never be used to enforce political ideology. Interest rates on loans should be well below market levels. They should be used to help the poorest in Third World countries most. Present policies help, all too often, the rich in the poor Third World at the expense of their poorer neighbours. These however are almost beyond hope with President Reagan in the USA and the present (1985) administration in the UK.

THE LAW OF THE SEA

The UN Conference on the Law of the Sea is another example of the rich world's bad treatment of the poorer three-quarters of the world's population. The poor countries attach great importance to the principle that deep sea bed mineral resources are the common heritage of mankind. This was the subject of long discussion involving private and collective exploitation, 'production limit per year' and so on. A compromise position had been apparently reached in 1979–80. In summer 1980 the Carter administration in the USA indicated it was willing to accept the text. Britain, and others, agreed. The new Reagan administration, however, in 1981 demanded the right to reconsider the matter. In 1982 the Reagan administration, despite new compromise proposals, rejected the Treaty — Britain then too rejected the text, also West Germany and a few others; but other EEC members accepted the Treaty, as did also **all the Commonwealth countries except Britain**.

The danger is that once an uncontrolled scramble to exploit deep sea minerals begins, the ecological damage done could be as bad or worse than that due to the destruction of trees. It is not people's need for essential food that strains earth's resources but other necessary requirements (such as fuel for cooking) and unnecessary 'market-created' wants. If and when these deep sea minerals are exploited they should be shared and used gradually. The required techniques for exploitation are not yet developed — fortunately.

THE BRANDT COMMISSION REPORTS

NORTH AND SOUTH: THE FIRST BRANDT REPORT, 1980

This report of an independent Commission on International Development was the result of their two year long deliberations. Willy Brandt was the Chairman of this 20 member Commission from various nations, half from the 'North', half from the 'South'; Edward Heath represented the UK. It was submitted to the United Nations in February 1980, and its findings and conclusions can be read in a 300 page book *North and South: a Programme for Survival*. The developed wealthy 'North' is here taken to also include Australia and New Zealand; the other nations, 'South', are the poorer, less developed ones.

The report describes the gross inequalities between 'North' and 'South'. The 'North', including Eastern Europe, has a quarter of the world's population and 80% of its income, consumes 85% of its oil and produces 90% of its manufactured goods. The 'North' is not yet half way to its aid target of 0.7% of GNP, but it is still increasing armament expenditure. The report suggests a tax on arms trade to finance international aid — an excellent idea but . . .

The cost of one tank could buy 1,000 classrooms — the cost of one jet fighter could provide 40,000 village pharmacies.

Mutual interest of 'North' and 'South' is a central theme of the report. It proposed that conventional financial and technical aid be increased by $30 billion per year, and oil prices stabilized. A more prosperous 'South' is seen as a potential market. The general trend is economic in the financial sense, rather than in the more reasonable social and ecological terms and the fact that the 'North's' dietary extravagances have got to change is only touched upon. For example 'the rich of the world could help to increase food supplies if they used less fertilizer for non-food purposes and also if they ate less meat; to produce one unit of meat protein uses up to eight units of vegetable protein, which could be consumed directly' . . . '3 to 8 kilograms of cereal to each kilogram of edible poultry . . . sufficient to supply a large proportion of the world's hungry people with cereal products' . . . 'such changes of habit may be distant'. Just how distant? one wonders.

'It [the report] does not question the economic forces and social structures, either in the North or South, which create and perpetuate poverty. Without such questioning the Commission's proposals . . . are of dubious value. As they stand they are more than likely to benefit the rich in poor countries at the expense of the poor in rich countries.' *New Internationalist* April 1980

The Brandt Report recommended greatly increased aid to the Third World, but before the report was debated in the House of Commons the Government had decided to further reduce our much too low aid programme.

TABLE 7: NET PUBLIC EXPENDITURE ON AID (UK)

	77/78	78/79	79/80	80/81	81/82	82/83	83/84	84/85	85/86	86/87
£m – cash	600	715	784	885	959	965	1,031	1,099	1,130	1,170
£m – constant 83/84 prices	1,125	1,214	1,138	1,084	1,067	1,008	1,031	1,047	1,027	1,013
As % of total government spending	1.05	1.09	1.02	0.95	0.92	0.85	0.86	0.87	0.86	0.86
As % of GNP	0.44	0.46	0.52	0.35	0.43	0.37	0.35			

The net aid spending for 1985/86 will thus be 2% down in real terms on 84/85, after inflation at 5% is taken into account, and 86/87 is planned to decline further in real terms.

Source WDM Dec. 84–Jan 85

COMMON CRISIS: THE SECOND BRANDT REPORT 1983

The introduction by Willy Brandt is dated December 1982 — two years after the first report. It gives an objective account of the present world situation and while not blaming the affluent ex-colonial nations for producing world poverty does reproach them for their lack of generosity and foresight.

It points out that 'the North-South Summit at Cancun, Mexico, in the fall of 1981 [proposed in the first report and which had aroused great anticipation] fell short of our expectations' and that the state of the Third World is worse now than it was then. It gives many specific instances of this. For example: African countries now, on average, import 8% to 9% of their food; the destruction of tree cover for fuel and its consequences; the alarming long term prospects for developing countries due to rapid population increase; that even when food surpluses are generated in the Third World their poor still go hungry; and so on. It also again contrasts the enormous sums of money spent on military purposes with those donated to real Third World aid.

There are eight pages of a Resume of Principal Proposals, the first five pages of which relate to finance. Many of the 35 proposals under this heading are rather technical and at times vague. They amount to saying that the IMF should be more generous with regard to special drawing rights and loan conditions etc; the rich developed world should be more generous with regard to aid ('a new commitment to reach the 0.7% of GNP target for official development assistance within five years'); and in general the rich nations should do far more than they have. They are worthy objectives but most unlikely to be implemented. Worse still, they are based on the false assumption that an economic system motivated by acquisitive gain and employing money lending can somehow cure the ills it has itself mainly caused.

Similar considerations also apply to the other 24 proposals under the headings: trade, food, energy, negotiating process. Of course the rich powerful developed countries should be less exacting with regard to trade, more inclined to help the food shortages and energy needs confronting poor countries; more flexible in negotiating; and so on — but they are very unlikely to be.

Again the assumption that trade is always mutually advantageous is false. 'According to a UNIDO study, developing countries could earn an extra $44 million (gross) per annum if their exports of seven major minerals had been taken up to the metal bar stage.' This of course applies to many other Third World products and is part of the poverty trap. Greed motivated commerce is neither generous or unexacting and trade between the rich, powerful, transnational dominated North and the very poor South will never be quite fair.

Long term prospects for developing countries are worrying (in FAO's words 'alarming'). 'To maintain present inadequate levels of demand imports of cereals would have to rise from an average 36.4 million tonnes in 1978/79 to 72 million in 1990 and 132 million tonnes by the end of the century . . . the financial implications add up to a situation which would be politically and economically unacceptable.'

The Second Brandt Report, like the first, is trapped in false and outmoded economic concepts. It is well motivated but the concept that all trade must be mutually beneficial is just not true. Cash crops, grown on land while the people starve, is one result of this trade. Trade between unequal partners will be to the disadvantage of the weaker one in nearly all cases. The position is complicated by the extreme inequalities of wealth within the poorer countries so that nothing gets grown unless it can be profitable to the over-rich land owners. A market economy is based on greed for money gain; one should not expect good to come from such a base.

> Capitalism is the extraordinary belief that the nastiest of men for the nastiest of motives will somehow work for the benefit of all.
>
> John Maynard Keynes

AID

THE EXAMPLE OF ETHIOPIA

Many millions of people in the poor countries are going to starve to death before our eyes. We will see them doing so on our television sets.

C. P. Snow, 1969

This came true for Ethiopia during winter 1984.

The profound promise of our era is that for the first time we have the technical capacity to free mankind from the scourge of hunger. Therefore today we must proclaim a bold objective: that within a decade no child will go to bed hungry, that no family will fear for its next day's bread, and that no human being's future and capacity will be stunted by malnutrition.

Dr Henry Kissinger, then US Secretary of State, at the World Food Conference in Rome, 1974

This promise has certainly not come true. In fact the number of hungry people has roughly doubled in the past decade (1974-1984). Over 500 million people today suffer from chronic malnutrition and the number of hungry people is continuously rising. It need not happen; it **could** be stopped.

In 1975 there were 54 countries unable to feed their existing population. Today (1984) that number is still rising. By the year 2000 it is feared it will have risen to 64 nations. The countries of south west Asia, Central America and Africa are most at risk.

Every minute of every day the EEC destroys 41 cauliflowers, 75 pounds of tomatoes, 438 peaches, 221 pounds of pears, 3170 pounds of apples, 51 pounds of mandarins, 1358 oranges, 1648 lemons.

Every minute of every day 30 people in the world die because of hunger or hunger-related diseases.

Hungry for Change Oxfam

In autumn 1984 public attention focussed on the plight of starving people in the drought smitten areas of Ethiopia and the public has responded generously to the film shown on television. In 1979 in a lesser famine the affluent nations gave Ethiopia its minimal handout of international aid (£5 per head, almost the lowest in the world) and agreed to set up a 60,000 tonne grain stockpile as a future insurance — not a tonne of which was delivered. The extent of Ethiopia's needs for food, trucks, medicine and so forth was regularly circulated worldwide and was updated every three months, and the present famine was anticipated. In December 1983 EEC members agreed to cut their 1984 aid in spite of their large store of surplus grain. Why? Ethiopia is one of the poorest nations (average income about £100 a year) and is riven by civil war which aggravates the effect of the drought.

According to the *Observer* (26/10/84) the Reverend Charles Elliott, until recently Director of Christian Aid, and Chairman of the Independent Group on British Aid (which produced the reports *Real Aid* in 1982 and *Aid is Not Enough* in 1984) suggests that Britain and the USA deliberately withheld aid from Ethiopia in the hope that a disastrous famine would bring down its Marxist government. The previous famine in Ethiopia, in 1973/74 when 200,000 people died, brought down the Emperor Haile Selassie.

While the current drought is the worst in Ethiopia since 1973/74 it is only part of a long term trend within a broad belt south of the Sahara, comprising the Sahel countries in the west (Senegal, Guinea Bissau, Mauritania, Mali, Burkina Faso, Niger, Chad), Sudan, and Ethiopia and Somalia in the east. Worse may still be to come. The facts have long been known but mainly ignored. At the start of 1984 the Reagan administration cut back the funds of the International Development Association, the main source to the poorest; while the British government cut back overseas aid when the Conservatives came to power in 1979. Britain's contribution to aid has never reached its target of 0.7% of its GNP; at 0.4% it is one of the lowest in Europe (see Table 7). It is difficult to see why — unless of course Dr Elliott is right.

In 1983 Britain spent £1,080 million on overseas aid, while during 1983/84 it earned more than £1,900 million from arms sales to the Third World.

Source: CAAT

FIGURE 15: AFRICAN COUNTRIES AFFECTED BY FAMINE

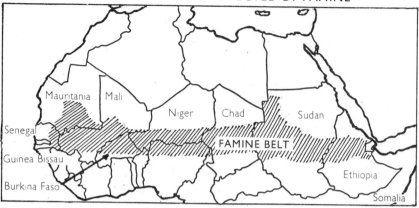

The United Nations Food and Agricultural Association identifies 24 countries in sub-Saharan Africa as 'most seriously affected' by food shortages. The World Bank predicts that over the next decade Africa could become so poor that 'between 65% and 80% of the people will be living below the poverty line'. Yet there is enough grain **alone** grown in the world to supply 3,000 calories a day per person — on average we each need 2,400 calories per day.

'AID IS NOT ENOUGH'

Aid, with its inadequacies, misdirection and misuse has been frequently referred to in previous sections. The heading of this section is the title of the Second Report (1984) of the Independent Group on British Aid. This is a group of seven, chaired by Professor Charles Elliott, all with full knowledge and experience in Third World matters, and the reports are very informative, balanced, searching and critical. Their First Report *Real Aid* was in 1982 when, to quote, 'we came to the conclusion that what should be its primary aim, to help the people of the receiving countries to help themselves by raising their productive capacity, was often subordinate to the aim of promoting purely British interests: the securing of contracts for British firms and the protection of jobs for British workers'.

In other words aid is all too often given 'with strings' attached:

a) Aid can be and is used, for example, to get rid of otherwise uncompetitive products; imports financed by aid are on average 30% higher in price than they would have been otherwise.

b) Aid can be used to open up a market. Once a poor country has imported an industrial product, partly financed by aid, it will almost certainly need further imports from the same source (e.g. spare parts and so on for imported plant or machines).

c) Aid is given or withheld on political considerations — which is one reason why the Third World has so many repressive, right wing governments.

But to return to *Aid is Not Enough*: 'There are many ways in which the policies which have been pursued by richer countries have made the problems of poor countries, and of poor people in poor countries, even worse than they would otherwise have been'. Some examples are given:

a) The Multi Fibre Arrangement (the means by which trade in textiles between rich countries and the poor is regulated). This agreement, imposed by the rich nations on the poor, places constraints on their exports of textiles and clothing, which can account for nearly one-third of their total manufactured exports, so such constraints hit underdeveloped countries hard.

b) The subsidized production of sugar (beet), for example, in the EEC has displaced Third World exports of this crop not only in EEC markets but in some Third World markets also.

c) A tight credit squeeze and high interest rates maintained by the rich countries for their own purposes has increased the cost of borrowing and debt repayments for Third World countries driving some to the verge of bankruptcy and so depressing still further their living standards.

d) Trade policy has often a **direct** effect on poor people. Customs and Excise officers throughout the EEC discriminate in a cavalier way against handloom goods. This simply robs women, the poor and the unemployed in the industrial sectors of Asia of a livelihood.

AID AND UNFAIR TRADE

In actual fact the rich North needs the poor South's resources far more than, in a free world, they would need the North's; but this is a world of mind-forged economic manacles.

Many raw materials vital to the rich world's industries are located only, or mainly, in the Third World while about 30% of the rich world's exports, and nearly 40% of US exports, go to the Third World. Some of the major multinationals make most of their profits in the Third World, while Third World countries are often heavily in debt to the rich world's banks and need their currency. This means the rich countries are able to fix the terms of all trade arrangements with the Third World and even 'play cat and mouse games' with them.

In 1975 the USA bought 1,000 million dollars worth of sugar from Brazil, but none in 1976. Instead it bought three times as much from the Philippines as it did in 1975. In 1976 the USA purchased 50% less Mexican cotton and 90% less Pakistani cotton than in 1975, but purchased four times as much Indian cotton as it did in 1975. This makes it possible for the USA to keep its costs down but makes a mess of any future plans in the poor country.

By 1982 world prices for the raw materials exported from the Third World were at their lowest for 50 years, which means it required much more exports to pay for the same quantity of oil. Also many poor countries depend on just one or two crops — nine African countries depend on just one crop for 70% of their income; 60% of Bangladesh's export earnings come from jute and jute products; 90% of Burundi's come from coffee. Thus the Third World countries find that having given up previously food-growing land for cash crops — a doubtful bargain — they are gradually getting less and less in return.

> ### Is Self Sufficiency in Food Necessary for World Peace?
>
> The Chinese maintained at the World Food Conference in Rome in 1974 that each country should be self sufficient, at least, in food in order that they can resist unfair bargaining in trade.
>
> Is this not a most important condition for world peace? But freedom from exploitation and non-indulgence in exploitation are equally vital.

THE MIS-FIT CAP OF THE EEC

It is clear that the UK and Europe as a whole could be self sufficient in food, if they were only prepared to do now what they will eventually have to do: change their diet to one less centred on animal products. This is true also for the USSR where too the animal food cult aggravates other economic difficulties (such as keeping up with NATO in the arms race). The Common Agricultural Policy (CAP) was intended to make the European Economic Community (EEC) self sufficient in food. It has not. It has made farming much more profitable and land owners and speculators rich by raising the price of land. It has wasted a great deal of public money, to create food gluts, and so led to deliberate destruction of food as well as its cheap sale to Russia. It has increased by its subsidies, the proportion of animal to vegetable food produced. Like other ill-conceived ideas it has been a disaster.

> In a written answer to the House of Commons on November 26th, Michael Jopling, Minister of Agriculture, said that expenditure by the Intervention Board for Agricultural Produce on storage and handling of intervention produced in the UK during 1983-84 came to £48.6 million.
>
> Timothy Raison, Minister for Overseas Development, said in a statement on January 5th that the UK allocation for disaster and refugee work during this current financial year amounts to £47 million.
>
> *Hungry for Change* Jan/Feb 1985

Entry to the EEC has been disastrous for the UK's trade. While most people are aware that we are now net importers of manufactured goods for the first time in at least 2000 years, they are not aware that most of the increase in imports come from EEC countries. In 1980 we had a surplus with the EEC in trade manufactured goods of £385 million (worth very much more at today's values). By 1984 this favourable balance had turned into a deficit of £8,864 million. This difference has cost at least a million jobs. Richard Body estimates it at 2 million.

The CAP takes two thirds of the EEC budget; about £9 billion in 1984. Its food mountains have become notorious. In Britain alone they include 55,600 tonnes of beef, 70,000 tonnes of bread-making wheat, 1,130,000 tonnes of feed wheat, 892,000 tonnes of barley. The dairy mountain consists of 164,000 tonnes of butter and 28,900 tonnes of skimmed milk powder. It costs £300 per minute just to keep Britain's stores of 'ood (WDM). Richard Body in *Farming in the Clouds* estimates the cost of UK expenditure on price support from 1955 to 1983 at £62 billion. The total land value of farm land in Britain he estimates at £64 billion — i.e. the taxpayer has all but purchased all the farmland. The cost is increasing continuously. He mentions how quite ordinary farmers in the mountains of Wales and the hills of Scotland are costing the taxpayer £50,000 a year to support. One farmer has an income of about £10,000 but the taxpayer in one way or another is paying out £75,000 a year for him. The book is a well researched case against the CAP.

To Third World countries in general the EEC must, like the USA, look like an economic conspiracy against them. It is after all a Customs Union euphemistically termed a Free Trade Area, and its levies are directed against outside producers. The EEC has a special arrangement with some 64 countries — the ACP (African, Caribbean and Pacific) states; it is the centrepiece of the EEC's development policy. The first Lome Convention was signed in 1975 and has been renegotiated since; it established aid and trade arrangements between the EEC and ACP countries. However less than one-eighth of the Third World's population live in the ACP countries. While the EEC has some arrangements with other poor countries the 12.5% of the Third World's population in ACP countries receive 80% of EEC aid. The agreements and arrangements and the way they are operated are of course complex and can only have cursory treatment here. The World Development Movement published four briefing papers on the EEC and the Third World in 1984, and the subject is dealt with in the books already referred to.

According to UNICEF five million children die every year because they have not been immunized. This would cost $5 a head, about £20 million per year. To support the CAP, Europe forks out £25 million per day.

Source: WDM

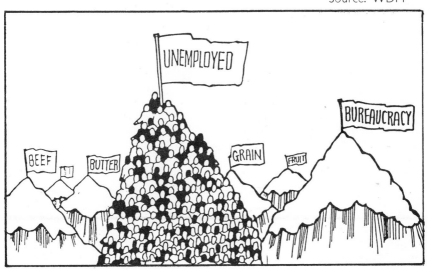

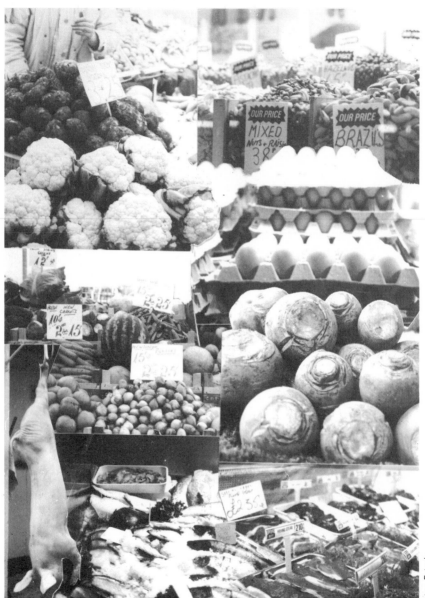

Monica Frisch

5 NUTRITION: FACT & FANCY

WHAT WE EAT

SOURCES OF PROTEIN AND ENERGY

Grains (wheat, barley, rye, oats, rice, corn (or maize), sorghum and some millets) together provide 50% of the world's protein and energy needs. If the grain converted to meat, milk, eggs, alcohol, etc. is added then 75% of the energy and protein needs are met from cultivated grain. (Animals used as converters of grain protein and other vegetable proteins are only 10% or so efficient.) Roots and tubers, potatoes, manioc, yams, taro, provide 8% of the energy and 5% of the protein of human consumption; peas, beans, nuts, oilseed — 5% of the energy and 12% of the protein; sugar — 9% of the energy and none of the protein; other fruits and vegetables 2% of the energy and 1% of the protein (SEE figure 16). These figures relate to the total energy (Calories) and proteins (tissue builders) supplied on a world scale by the foods mentioned — not to their relative merits.

There is however more to nutrition than calories and proteins — vitamins, mineral matter etc. are all involved. The human animal relies on 11 species of plant for 80% of its food. In a lifetime of say 70 years a human animal consumes about 20 or 30 tonnes of food; including in the rich world the edible parts of 8 cattle, 36 sheep, 36 pigs and 550 poultry. We eat 5 or 6 times our own weight in a year.

Smaller animals consume even more proportionally — a tonne of mice eats much more than a tonne of elephant, round about 50 or 60 times as much. These figures make clear the waste (in nitrates, phosphates, potash (NKP) etc.) involved in depositing human sewage in sea and rivers — or that involved in factory farming where this may be done with animal muck also. (SEE also 'the muck and magic fallacy').

FIGURE 16: WORLD SOURCES OF PROTEIN AND ENERGY IN THE HUMAN DIET

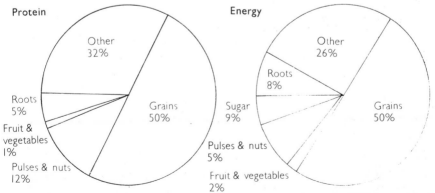

These diagrams are derived from figures given in *Scientific American* September 1976. It is assumed that 'other' includes fish, meat, eggs, dairy produce, alcohol etc.

CHOICE AND PERSUASION

Like other omnivores humans can live on a variety of diets. While most are mainly dictated by nature and necessity some are bizarre, like the Chinese consumption of birds' nests (including the adhesive ingredients, birds' saliva and excreta) — or the inexplicable outbreaks of soil eating in states around the lower part of the Missisippi. Travellers who have been entertained by Kurdish tribesmen can tell of their experience — or dread of — being presented, as a delicacy, with the eyeball of a goat, which a dirty hand and arm had extracted from the bowl in which most of the carcase had been boiled. The lucky recipient was expected to eat this with relish, and also to show his general appreciation by belching loudly at the end of the meal.

The diet of Eskimos, almost or entirely meat by necessity, is barely adequate. A photo, taken in 1955 (in the *Scientific American* September 1976) shows a pregnant Caribou Eskimo chewing a pile of caribou bones to extract the last scraps of the nutrient-rich marrow. These people lived in Canadian North West territories and depended entirely on the caribou, a large reindeer, for their food. In the late 1950s the caribou changed their migration route with disastrous results for these Eskimos. In 1960 the Canadian government airlifted the survivors to the coast where they mixed with other Eskimos and went to work in a nickel mine.

There are also the matters of knowledge, habit and custom. The Australian explorers Burke and Wills starved to death in an environment and in circumstances where an aborigine would have lived in comfort and an experienced explorer, like Sturt, would have managed easily. An African tribe kept cattle and used only the blood and milk, discarding the flesh — while Kosher meat must be quite free from blood.

G.B. Shaw, in one of his long prefaces, tells of a widow with a young family who, although poor, nevertheless contrived to keep herself and family well nourished, while near famine conditions prevailed; no one knew how. Eventually when pressed she reluctantly and tearfully confessed to the priest that at dawn she and her children went out into the country and collected all the snails they could find, which they later cooked and ate. That she should feel guilty about this is a strong indication of the kind of mental conditioning to which we are all subject from the cradle to the grave, even if we are not usually aware of it.

'People have never had freedom of choice in nutrition. With the best of intentions their parents misled them in their youth and with more questionable motives advertisers misled them in adult life'.

N W Pirie

ESSENTIALS OF HUMAN NUTRITION

All food provides the body with energy — calories — but a healthy diet requires adequate amounts of the various nutrients as well as sufficient calories. Calories alone may prevent starvation but not malnutrition and indeed can lead to problems of obesity. A healthy diet must be a balanced diet, with the right amounts of the various nutrients. Particularly with vitamins and minerals the proportions of each nutrient is important to enable the body to make the most of the nutrition it is getting. The types of nutrients the body requires are listed below.

PROTEINS
Body builders; repair tissues

Proteins are nitrogen containing compounds made up of amino acids. Most foods contain some protein.

CARBOHYDRATES
Provide energy (Calories)

Contain carbon, hydrogen and oxygen (but no nitrogen) — hydrogen and oxygen in the same proportions as in water. Excess carbohydrates can be converted into fats by human bodies inclined that way.

FATS
Provide energy that can be stored

In dry climates water can be stored in conjunction with fat, as in the camel's hump or the extra large buttocks of African bushmen.

VITAMINS
Absolutely essential to health, though only small amounts required.

Deficits produce diseases or weaknesses e.g. scurvy due to lack of vitamin C; rickets: lack of vitamin D; anaemia: lack of vitamin B12.

MINERALS
A great many are needed in varying quantities

Lack of calcium causes rickets and weak bones and teeth for example.

FIBRE
Roughage

Lack causes constipation and intestinal problems.

WATER
Most essential as the body is mainly water

No problem as long as it is pure, and there is an adequate supply.

Proteins, carbohydrates, fats, all contain the chemical elements, carbon, hydrogen and oxygen, but only proteins contain nitrogen. Carbohydrates provide energy (measured in Calories or K joules), but proteins are essential for tissue replacement and new growth. Sugar is pure carbohydrate and provides only calories, but many foods like potato and bread provide considerable quantities of protein and are not only carbohydrates.

PROTEINS

Protein is found not only in foods considered protein foods but also in many others. Our bodies are 18% to 20% protein by weight. Skin, hair, cartilage and muscles, are made up largely of fibrous proteins. Body regulators like hormones and enzymes are proteins; haemoglobin (the oxygen carrying molecule in the blood) is built of protein.

Amino Acids

Proteins are compounds made up of amino acids. Different protein foods contain different proportions of the 20 or so amino acids. When eaten proteins are broken down into amino acids and built up again into the unique proteins for the different parts of the body — unique even for each particular person. Of the 20 or so amino acids 8 or 9 are considered **essential** and cannot be synthesized by the body from other amino acids.

The position is complicated but a combination of different protein foods eaten **together** is much more satisfactory than relying on just one protein source (as explained in the next section). Combining foods to produce a better amino acid balance is termed 'complementing' them. The subject is dealt with fully in *Diet for a Small Planet* which also gives recipes based on the use of complementary protein combinations. A varied diet of different protein foods can provide all that is required; neither meat nor dairy produce need be included.

Protein Complementarity

FIGURE 17: PROTEIN COMPLEMENTARITY

Amount of essential amino acids as % of levels in WHO standard reference protein

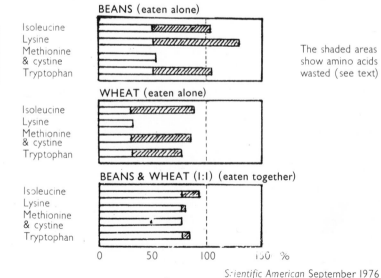

The five animo acids indicated in the diagram (fig. 17) are the most critical of the eight or nine essential amino acids. The body building and tissue repair value of any protein eaten alone, at one meal, depends on the amount of the weakest amino acid present (e.g. methionine and cystine in beans, lysine in wheat). Excess of the other amino acids results in their use as fuel only, like carbohydrates, so that the shaded portions of the amino acids shown are waste as far as tissue building and repair are concerned.

The **proportion** of protein eaten which is thus wasted is much less in the bean-wheat combination than in either eaten separately. The 100% dotted line in the diagrams represents the amino acid of a standard reference protein chosen by the United Nations World Health Organization (WHO) as best meeting human needs. Its use here is merely as a standard since the actual amount of each amino acid consumed would depend on the total quantity of the food eaten: 110 grammes of the bean-wheat combination would be about the same as 75 grammes of egg. (Egg approximates closely to the WHO standard protein.) Grain and pulse foods are generally good complementary pairs and combinations like beans on toast are found in many cultures.

The WHO has given the following weights necessary to provide the daily requirements of the eight essential amino acids.

Isoleucine	700 mg	Leucine	1100 mg
Lysine	800 mg	Methionine	400 mg
Phenylalanine	300 mg	Threonine	500 mg
Valine	800 mg	Tryptophan	250 mg

Cystine and methionine are the sulphur containing amino acids.

To obtain the necessary quantity of each and all of these one would need to eat about 500g of peas, 1147g of potatoes, 44g of soyflour, 92g of meat or drink half a litre of milk. Combining and complementing the protein foods consumed during a meal very considerably reduces these amounts except in the cases of meat, soyflour and milk. The old notion of meat as first class protein is now generally discarded. Soya beans when thoroughly cooked to make them digestible are better; so is precooked soyflour and textured vegetable protein (TVP). TVP like other soya products has a very high nutritional value (vitamin B12 has been added and it contains other B vitamins also). Some has been given various meat and other flavours, and it can be used in a variety of recipes. The meat flavours may fail to satisfy meat eaters while offending vegetarians. Sosmix and Burgamix, more recent soya products, are easier to use. They make good rissoles and similar products. These products are not robbing the Third World, as a review of the first edition of this book suggested. The USA is the largest grower of soya beans in the world and exports about 50% of its crop. There is no overall shortage of protein in the USA. Soya beans have been grown as a source of raw material for plastic knobs and pieces for cars and much is fed to animals. When as in the UK and other over developed countries imported soya beans and peanuts from poor countries where food shortage is rife are fed to animals for an average 10% or so protein return it is nothing less than a crime.

TABLE 8: AMOUNTS OF PROTEIN & FATS IN FOOD AS PURCHASED

	Protein	Fat		Protein	Fat
Cheddar cheese	25.4%	34.5%	Soya (dry)	40.3%	23.5%
Chicken	20.8%	6.7%	Peanuts	28.1%	49.0%
Beef	18.1%	17.1%	Lentils (dry)	23.8%	trace
Fish (steamed cod)	17.4%	0.7%	Almonds	20.5%	53.5%
Bacon	15.8%	40.5%	Flour	12.2%	2.4%
Eggs	10.9%	12.3%	Bread wheat	9.6%	3.1%

NOTE: figures of this kind vary considerably from source to source

MAFF Manual of Nutrition, The Law and the Loaf

FATS AND OILS

While some fat and oil is essential it is now generally agreed that those eating a Western type diet consume too much fat and oil, especially saturated fats, and should try to eat less. Edible oils and fats contain carbon, hydrogen and very little oxygen and are compounds of glycerol (glycerine) and fatty acids. Mineral oils like medicinal paraffin are not desirable in foods. Saturated fats (saturated with hydrogen) in excess may contribute to heart disease. Oils are sometimes saturated to turn them into solid fats (hydrogenation) as in margarine manufacture. Unsaturated fats and oils have a valuable role to play in human metabolism and should preferably predominate over the saturated kinds. In general animal products contain more saturated fats while vegetable products contain more unsaturated oils. In vegetable oils like soya oil, sunflower seed oil and maize oil, the polyunsaturated ingredients predominate. A few vegetable fats like coconut butter are little better than animal fats in this respect. Some vegetable margarines indicate on the package the degree of unsaturated oils they contain. This is too complex a topic to be dealt with fully here; it is connected with the concentration of cholesterol in the blood plasma and the risk of a coronary heart attack.

VITAMINS

Vitamins and a number of inorganic elements (about 20) are also necessary. A varied diet, including fresh fruit and vegetables, usually provides these and deficiency effects today are rare in Britain, though this was not the case in the past. Before 1912 nothing definite was known about vitamins and even now knowledge may not be complete; although in 1747 a Scottish naval surgeon, James Lind, on HMS Salisbury, two centuries ahead of his time, showed that a small ration of oranges or lemons prevented and cured scurvy (now known to be due to a deficiency of vitamin C). There is some evidence that high doses of some vitamins, such as vitamin C, can be used medicinally to prevent or cure certain ailments, but it should be noted that others are toxic in high doses.

TABLE 9: VEGETARIAN SOURCES OF VITAMINS

Vitamin A   Insoluble in water, soluble in oils and fats. Vitamin A as carotene is added to most margarines. It is not affected by cooking. Deficiency effects such as poor vision in the dark are rare in the UK.

Sources: Carrots, butter, milk, eggs, green plants, spinach, cabbage, lettuce, brussels sprouts, peas, dried apricots, tomatoes, prunes.

Vitamin B group A complex of about 12 different substances.

B1   Thiamine (aneurine). Soluble in water, destroyed in cooking. Deficiency effects: growth check, depression, neuritis, beri beri. Daily need about 1 mg.

B2   Riboflavin. Water soluble, not easily destroyed by cooking. Deficiency causes sores in mouth and on tongue. Daily need about 1.5 mg.

B5   Niacin (nicotinic acid). Water soluble, not destroyed by cooking. Lack causes rough skin, sore tongue, diarrhoea, mental symptoms, pellagra. Daily need about 12 mg.

Sources: B1, B2 and B5 are in brewer's yeast, Marmite, Yeastrel, Barmene, Tastex, etc, cheese, eggs, wholemeal bread, oatmeal, peas, beans, nuts, potatoes, beer, wheatgerm (Bemax and Froment).

B12   Cobalamins (hydroxycobalamins). Lack causes pernicious anaemia and degeneration of the spinal cord. (See note on B12).

M   Folic acid (folacin). This works in close relationship with B12 and deficiencies again result in anaemia and degeneration of the nervous system.

Sources: It is found in dried baker's yeast as well as in vegetables.

Vitamin C   Ascorbic acid. Soluble in water, not in fats. Boiled out in cooking. Lack causes sub-scurvy — laziness, gloom, irritability, slow healing of wounds.

Sources: Rose hips, blackcurrrants, brussels sprouts, sprouting broccoli, cabbage, watercress, oranges, lemons, grapefruit, new potatoes, lettuce, carrots, etc.

Vitamin D   Calciferol. Soluble in fats, insoluble in water. Controls the absorption of calcium and phosphorus to form teeth and bones.

Sources: Food and sunlight. Foods: eggs, butter, cheeses, milk, fortified margarine.

Vitamins A, D and B12 are stored in the liver — not lost in urine as other B vitamins and vitamin C are.

There are other B vitamins (not listed here) whose deficiency are extremely unlikely. Other vitamins not listed here include E (anti-toxic) and K (blood clotting vitamin) and are found in green vegetables, wheatgerm etc.

Note on vitamin B12

B12 is produced by micro-organisms. In humans it is produced by bacteria in the large intestine but too far down the digestive tract to be of use of us. So humans have to get it from other sources.

B12 is not, as previously thought, exclusive to liver and meat, milk, cheese, and eggs. Yeast extracts, like Barmene and Tastex, also contain B12. It is also produced by the action of some strains of bacteria in the soil and worm casts are rich in B12 due to bacteria in the worm's digestive tract. Small amounts are found on some plants due to bacterial contamination and in some seeds and seaweed. 50g to 100g of laverbread or dulse (not contaminated by sewage) would provide the daily requirements of B12.

B12 can be produced by various kinds of mould culture. It is an important by-product of the process of preparing the antibiotic streptomycin. It can therefore by used to fortify plant milk and other vegan foods. Plamil brand soya milks contain B12 — 100 ml of this undiluted milk would provide daily human requirements. B12 is stored in the liver, so deficiency symptoms may not immediately follow deprivation. Daily requirement, though essential, is very small, 1 to 2 micrograms (millionth of a gramme); the quantity that can be absorbed daily is only two or three times as great. More about this vitamin is given in a one page leaflet *Vegan Compost and Vitamin B12*, in *Vegan Nutrition* and in the larger book *Vegetarian Nutrition*. The other B vitamins, including folic acid, are abundant in food of plant origin as well as in animal products.

INORGANIC ELEMENTS

The body obtains about 20 elements or minerals from food and their importance is being increasingly recognized. New evidence is linking mineral deficiencies with a number of ailments. They are needed in balanced proportions and usually a varied diet will supply them in the right quantities and proportions. The main elements are sodium, potassium, calcium, phosphorus, iodine and iron. Trace elements include magnesium, sulphur, fluorine, cobalt and zinc. Rich sources of trace elements include kelp and other seaweeds, nuts, and seeds such as sesame and sunflower.

For further information see the publications on nutrition listed at the end of this book.

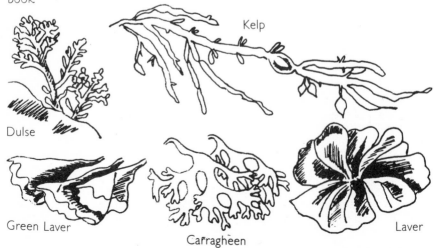

Kelp

Dulse

Green Laver

Carragheen

Laver

WHAT DOES THE UNITED KINGDOM EAT?

TABLE I0: AVERAGE WEEKLY EXPENDITURE ON FOOD
(pence per head per week)

	1982		1977	
Meat	255	31.6%	178	34.9%
Fish	36	4.5%	20	3.9%
Cheese	28	3.5%	15	2.9%
Eggs	20	2.5%	15	2.9%
Milk	91	11.3%	53	10.4%
Bread	49	6.1%	30	5.9%
Fats	33	4.1%	24	4.7%
Fruit	48	6.0%	29	5.7%
Potatoes & vegetables	95	11.8%	52	10.2%
Cereals	76	9.4%	36	7.1%
Sugar & preserves	18	2.2%	13	2.6%
Tea, coffee, etc.	28	3.5%	21	4.1%
Sundry	29	3.5%	24	4.7%

Average: total/head/week   £8.06   £5.I0

Source: MAFF National Food Surveys 1978 and 1984

HOW DOES THIS COMPARE WITH THE PAST?

TABLE II: FOOD CONSUMPTION IN THE UK
(in pounds weight per head per year)

	1880	1909/13	1924/8	1941	1950	1960	1970	1980
Milk (pints)	213	219	217	265	347	319	311	265
Meat*	92	136	135	105	119	145	158	186
Cheese	8	7	9	8	10	10	12	13
Fish	18	41	41	16	22	19	20	20
Eggs	11	16	15	25	31	33	35	28
Butter	12	16	16	10	17	18	19	13
Margarine	0	6	12	18	17	15	12	15
Other fats	-	4	6	18	19	22	26	24
Sugar	64	79	87	67	83	112	106	72
Potatoes	296	208	194	188	246	224	226	198
Other vegetables**	-	83	106	123	132	133	140	153
Fruit & nuts	-	69	118	30	86	106	112	102
Wheat flour	280	211	198	237	206	166	146	142
Other cereals	-	26	16	20	17	14	17	16

* carcase weights; includes bacon, ham, poultry
** includes pulses and tomatoes

Source: Changing Food Habits in the UK; MAFF

MALNUTRITION IN BRITAIN

Undernourishment is mainly a thing of the past, due usually to sheer poverty, reinforced by ignorance of food values and commercial conditioning. In 1917 half of Britain's children were prone to rickets. When conscription was brought in, in 1916, three out of every nine men of military age were quite fit and healthy, two were in some respect inferior, three were incapable of more than a very moderate degree of exertion (physical wrecks) and one was a chronic invalid. In spite of the Depression between the Wars there was a considerable improvement in average health, but Boyd Orr's survey *Food, Health and Income* (1936) showed that all was far from well especially among the poorer sections.

In 1935, 62% of volunteers for the army were turned down on medical grounds. In the Second World War (1939–45) extensive efforts were made to increase agricultural output. By 1944 wheat output had increased by 90%, potatoes by nearly as much, vegetables by 45%, sugar beet by 19% and output of barley and oats doubled. Government food subsidies kept food prices down; 'British Restaurants', at first an emergency service in blitzed areas, continued to supply cheap and satisfactory meals. Agriculture has not since been neglected as it was before the First World War and to a lesser degree between the two Wars — nutrition and health have in general remained good. Average health was at its highest during the last War, in spite of shortages, or even perhaps partly because of them. Foods during that period were more natural — bread was nearer to whole grain, meat consumption was low, there were less highly refined foods and others whose nutritional value had been reduced in manufacture; there was less overeating and less sugar and fat were consumed.

Undernourishment depends on real poverty, which is a consequence of an extremely uneven distribution of wealth. When and where the community as a whole is relatively affluent extreme differences of wealth within it have less serious effects on nutrition. Britain, Europe, Japan and even the USA have probably passed their apogee of affluence — future economic expansion, increased productivity, etc. are really impossible — so malnutrition may well reappear in these countries as it did during the depression years of the 1920s and 1930s. Indeed there are indications that in Britain it is on the way. A MORI poll for London Weekend Television in 1982 estimated that more than seven million people went without food at some time in the year through lack of money. An article (*Sunday Times Magazine* 10/11/85) refers to an indepth survey of the Food Policy Unit of Manchester Polytechnic and gives four examples of daily diets (ages 17 to 79). They are clearly quite inadequate whether due to poverty or lack of nutritional information. Packets of potato crisps are most expensive forms of nutrition and sundry choc bars are little better. The very poor are tempted to go for satisfying, filling 'junk' foods.

In the UK the richest 5% own nearly half the personal capital wealth and the richest 1% own about a quarter thereof. There are a growing number of people without enough income to ensure adequate necessities and nutrition. Young children, the elderly, and pregnant women are especially likely to suffer from an inadequate diet.

There is another form of malnutrition which is common in Britain: over-nutrition. Nearly half the population are slightly to excessively overweight and their general health suffers in consequence. Britain has been described as 'a nation of constipated, toothless fatties'. This of course applies also the the USA and other affluent countries, and to the rich minorities in the Third World. Even the very poor can sometimes be obese although undernourished as a cheap inadequate diet can be fattening.

Dangerous conditions correlated with excessive body fat include diabetes, gallstones and degenerative diseases of the kidney, heart and arteries; while those related to excessive weight include arthritis (undue strain on joints), hernia, varicose veins, and broken bones. A slightly defective heart which could manage with a normal body weight might well fail to cope with excess body weight.

What we eat is a matter of habit conditioned by persistent persuasion. Advertising pressures during the last century have had a powerful influence. White bread and breakfast cereals have replaced wholegrain bread. Food more and more tends to come in cardboard packages or tins, and to be less natural, so we pay more for less nutritional value. However there is now a trend back towards 'natural' 'wholefoods'. Needless to say commercial interests have jumped on the bandwagon and are selling wholefoods. For example the Holland and Barratt health food chain is owned by Booker McConnell, a multinational whose other interests include engineering, pharmaceuticals and the Budgen chain of supermarkets. Commerciogenic malnutrition is not confined to the Third World, though its effects now are far worse there.

> Nothing more strongly arouses our disgust than cannibalism, yet we make the same impression on Buddhists and vegetarians, for we feed on babies, though not our own.
>
> Robert Louis Stevenson
>
> I have no doubt it is part of the destiny of the human race . . . to leave off eating animals.
>
> H D Thoreau

FOOD PACKAGING AND ADDITIVES

The elaborate packaging of food shows an outlook that regards food as a profit-maker and job provider, in that order, rather than as an essential to life and health. In some cases the package can cost as much or more than the food it contains, while nutritional values are often greatly diminished in food manufacture.

There is a legal obligation for food manufacturers to list the ingredients, including additives, on the tin or package. They are worth reading even if they are often vague. Some additives may adversely affect some people; for example monosodium glutamate is used to enhance natural flavours but can bring a few people out in rashes or flushes. Nitrates and nitrites are added to preserved meat; nitrites to prevent botulism (actually they merely retard it and so increase the shelf life of the cured meat). Nitrates convert to nitrites in the human gut and later to nitrosamines which are carcinogens.

There are lists of prohibited and permitted additives; but the USA list for example bans some permitted in the UK and allows the use of some prohibited in the UK — so just how reliable are the prohibitions? A variety of substances have been used to bleach flour: alum, ammonia, gypsum, nitrogen trichloride (agene). The last, in 1947 was found to produce hysteria in dogs. Its use was soon prohibited. Chalk is added to white bread as a source of calcium but its nutritional value is doubtful.

In broiler chickens and meat growth promoting substances like hormones, antibiotics, copper and arsenic, may still be present. Poultry and other meat may contain drug resistant bacteria; this could result in causing those who consumed such meat, and subsequently picked up a germ, to be unresponsive to the usual antibiotic treatment.

The vast majority of food additives are for the manufacturers' convenience, to ease processing and storage, or to enhance appearance. They rarely have any nutritional value and in many cases are positively harmful. There are exceptions; as well as added vitamins others may be beneficial. Lecithin, used as an emulsifier, could incidently help in reducing cholesterol.

Fresh food, free from pesticides etc. is best. In processed foods there are far too many artificial colours and artificial flavours. They could and should be eliminated while the preservatives should be reduced in number and quantity.

The MAFF has issued a free booklet _Look at the Label_ about the ingredients listed on food packages for sale. It lists some 172 substances, denoted by E numbers (used in EEC countries) which can be used as alternatives to their specific names, but fails to give any information about their origin or nature. The book _E for Additives_ by Maurice Hanssen, gives full information about these substances. There is a glossary of E numbers with other useful information about common food additives and contaminants and lists of food and drink etc. of interest to vegetarians and vegans in _The 1985/86 International Vegetarian Handbook_. This also gives vegetarian restaurants, hotels, etc. in the UK and Europe. See also booklist.

HOW IMPORTANT IS BREAD?

Bread is an outstanding example of a natural product, damaged by commercial interests and perverted public taste. Natural vitamins are removed in milling together with a number of mineral elements. A good account of this is given in _The Law and the Loaf_. Harvey Day's book _About Bread_ deals more with the US position than the UK one.

Bread provides the average person in the UK today with 15% of energy and 12% of protein intake. In the past, when it was called the staff of life, it provided much more. The story of bread is a tragedy of errors. In the wheat grain nature has provided (as in other seeds and embryos) the maximum nutrition in a small space — life in the seed passes through the gate of nutrition. The human incapacity, especially where profit is involved, to leave well alone has resulted in that devitalised product, white bread — every day in the UK millions of white sliced loaves are consumed. The false notion that white bread is more digestible and hence better than wholemeal goes back for centuries — fortunately for a long period the poorer sections of the community were helped by the fact that white bread was more expensive.

FIGURE 18: A WHEAT GRAIN

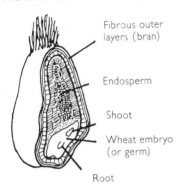

Fibrous outer layers (bran)

Endosperm

Shoot

Wheat embryo (or germ)

Root

In the old stone-grinding process the embryo or germ was retained with the inner endosperm.

In modern (from the second half of the 19th century) steel roller milling to produce white flour the germ is removed with the bran. The wheat germ contains most of the vitamins of the B group, and mineral elements, while the bran supplies valuable roughage.

In the nineteenth century the influx of cheaper grain from North America and the growth of roller milling made it possible to separate the germ and the endosperm (white central part) from the bran (SEE figure 16). White flour is made from the endosperm (70% of the whole grain). The germ and the bran make up the 30% removed. The removed portion contains vitamins, especially those of the B complex, and various mineral elements — it is a very considerable nutritional loss. The removed 30% is worth £86 million per year as animal feed and for pet food. Unground grain is comparatively easy to store; white flour keeps well, but wholegrain flour, because of the oils from the germ, does not keep so well.

There is a great difference between wholesale world wheat prices and the price of flour. The EEC levy (due to the CAP) and the near monopoly in the milling industry (three transnational firms control 80% of UK flour production) explain why. The first results in over-production (intervention purchase and storage by the EEC) and the second, like all monopolies, means high profits. Those who bake their own bread may prefer flour from the non-monopoly 20% as it is generally freer from additives. Flour from home grown wheat has less gluten and does not rise as well as that from imported wheat and is more inclined to crumble. Some flour made from home grown wheat has some imported grain flour added for this reason.

In 1976 the Vegetarian Society began its Campaign for Real Bread (CAMREB) on the lines of CAMRA (the Campaign for Real Ale) as part of its Green Plan for greater UK self-sufficiency in food, fuels and timber. Such campaigns are well worth while. Fortunately far more wholegrain bread is now being produced commercially than was the case even six or ten years ago, even if it is by no means free from additives.

FIGURE 19: WHITE AND WHOLE GRAIN BREAD

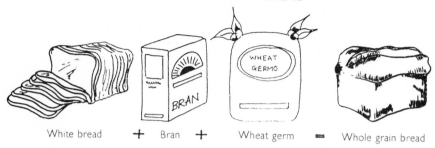

| White bread | + | Bran | + | Wheat germ | = | Whole grain bread |

Equal nutrition maybe; but cost of separate nutrients much greater than the equivalent quantity of wholegrain bread.

White bread is 70% of the whole grain. The bran and wheat germ (30%) are called 'wheat offal' in the trade. They contain, mainly in the wheat germ, the B vitamins and mineral elements of high nutritional value. Some wheatgerm is sold at an inflated price in packets in health food shops, also some of the bran as 'All Bran' and so on, but most wheat offal goes for animal fodder and pet food.

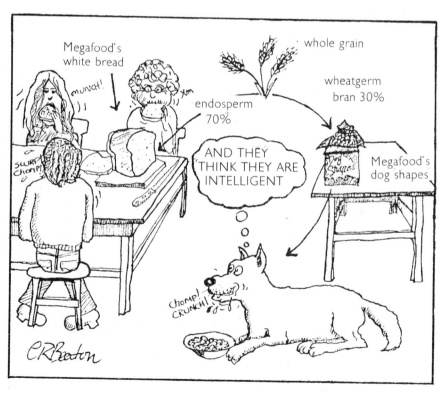

FIGURE 20: EMMER WHEAT

Emmer was the common wheat of Egypt until Alexander the Great conquered the country in 331 BC when it was replaced by 'bread wheat'. For some millenia emmer was a most successful and valuable crop. A later mutant emmer is the ancestor of modern macaroni wheats. 'Bread wheat' is a cross between the later mutant emmer (or macaroni wheat) and goat grass. it arose much later than emmer and modern wheats are mainly derived from it. The FAO of the United Nations preserves genetic banks of wheat seeds, including emmers, as sources for possible future strains.

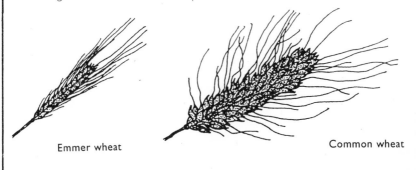

Emmer wheat   Common wheat

THE VEGAN DIET

There are many reasons why people go vegan (and vegetarian).

a) Simple revulsion to meat and flesh foods — even very young children of five or six sometimes show this;

b) Objection to the cruelty involved — factory farming is most disgusting but so is conventional dairy farming. The calf is taken from its mother at birth to the distress of both, for a food which is harmful and unnatural. ('Milk is a major killer. It is a nonsense to give it to children in school' Sir Douglas Black, President of the BMA, according to the Sunday Times 12/6/84.) A modern cow leads a hell of a life: 9 months pregnant, 9 months lactating, and 6 months both; a calf every year. When at last she fails she is sent to the abattoir as a final reward.

c) To improve one's health;

d) Ecological — an animal product diet requires much more land per person to produce it than one which uses only plant products. If all, or most, people became vegan there would be land to spare which could be used for other purposes. The overdeveloped world would not need to rob (by unfair trade) the poor world of vital food. We would need much less fertilizer also. There are some who become vegan because they see that our animal centred diet is doing, and can only do, great damage to the poor countries.

SOME VEGETARIAN AND VEGAN RECIPES

Many common dishes are vegetarian and some are also vegan. While for example macaroni cheese, pizza, cheese and egg salads are vegetarian, beans on toast and any salad without animal or fish products are vegan also. A pizza can be made using a soya 'cheese' (made from soya flour and vegetarian margarine) while many conventional meat dishes can easily be converted to vegan ones by simple substitution of lentils, nuts or soya products (e.g. TVP) for the meat. There are many vegetarian and vegan recipe books available (see list at the end of this book). A visit to a health food store reveals some of the vegan products available.

There is no need to make a burden of a vegan diet. There are many simple alternatives to meat or dairy products, such as beans, lentils and soya beans (an excellent inexpensive source of protein). Many beans need soaking and lentils also are better soaked.

While vegetarianism is a welcome first step, its value as a means of reducing cruelty and helping the world's poor and reducing ecological damage is at best limited. Veganism is the proper goal (SEE previous section).

Lentil Hot Pot

8oz. red lentils	I dessertsp. yeast extract (e.g. Marmite)
I lb. potatoes	¾ pint warm water
3 onions	I tsp. dried herbs
2oz. margarine	Seasoning to taste

Put layers of lentils, sliced potatoes and sliced onions into an oven dish, seasoning between layers and finishing with potatoes. Dissolve yeast extract in the warm water and pour over. Dot with margarine and cover. Bake in a moderate oven for about one hour, or until tender, and brown off without lid. Serve with green vegetables.

* If vegan margarine (containing no dairy products) is used this dish is vegan.

Risotto

2 tablesp. oil	I tsp. yeast extract
I medium onion	Bouquet garni or herbs to taste
I cup brown rice	¼ lb. mushrooms
2 cups water	2oz. sunflower seeds
½ red pepper	

Fry chopped onion in the oil to soften. Add rice and cook for several seconds, turning with a fork. Add hot water in which the yeast extract has been dissolved and herbs. Bring to the boil and simmer gently. After ½ hour add the chopped mushrooms and simmer for a further 20-25 minutes, until the rice is cooked. Season to taste, add the sunflower seeds and chopped pepper.

* This dish is vegan. It can be varied by adding more or different vegetables (e.g. peas, sweetcorn, tomatoes).

6 FOOD, ECOLOGY AND AGRICULTURE

WHAT IS THE SOURCE OF ENERGY IN FOOD?

Plants are the source of all food. Animal products are second hand ones, derived from plants by very inefficient means. Sunlight is the source of the energy (calories) in food, as it is also of the energy in fossil fuels (coal, gas, oil). Green plants capture solar energy with an efficiency of 15% to 22%, but this captured energy is only 1% of the total solar energy reaching the earth. The bulk of a plant, over 97%, comes from air and water; a tree is not, as G. K. Chesterton said, a piece of earth thrust upwards, but rather air and water turned solid. The carbon in a plant comes from the carbon dioxide in the air, the hydrogen and oxygen from water drawn up with the sap. Nitrogen, an essential constituent of proteins, can only be obtained from soluble substances in the soil, although four-fifths of the air is nitrogen. Nitrogen forms about 2% of the dry matter of a plant; phosphorus about 0.2%.

The annual production of fixed carbon by green plants, on land and in the sea, is about 150 billion tonnes; human consumption about 0.42 billion tonnes/year, about 570 kilogrammes per head. If all the energy captured by plants could be directed to human needs the world could support 280 times its present population.

CARBON CYCLE

The carbon cycle is the basis of carbohydrate and all food production.

Plants use carbon dioxide in the air, and water from the soil, to produce carbohydrates and oxygen. The energy for this process comes from sunlight which is absorbed by the chlorophyll (green colouring) in the leaves. This process is called photosynthesis.

FIGURE 21: CARBON CYCLE   FIGURE 22: NITROGEN CYCLE

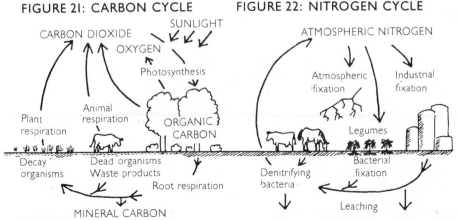

Animals burn up carbohydrates and through respiration change oxygen back to carbon dioxide. Plants respire too, but in the light produce more oxygen by photosynthesis than they consume. The decay of leaves and other vegetable and animal matter in the soil produces humus rich in organic carbon — a most valuable addition.

NITROGEN CYCLE

The nitrogen cycle is the basis of protein formation, by 'fixing' nitrogen in a form which can be used.

Atmospheric nitrogen can be converted into water soluble substances, by bacterial action (particularly the bacteria associated with the roots of legumes), by industrial chemical processes, and a small amount by the action of lightning. Fixed nitrogen can be absorbed by plants and used to convert carbohydrates into proteins. The nitrogen is freed again as plants rot and animals excrete.

TOTAL NUTRIENT CYCLE
FIGURE 23: THE NUTRIENT CYCLE

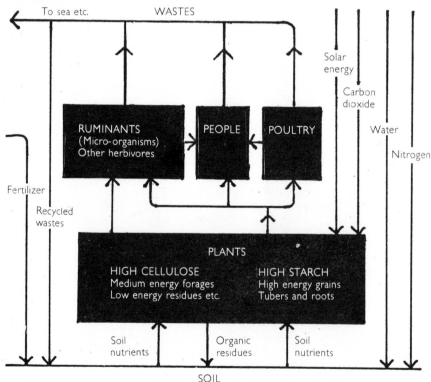

As well as carbon and nitrogen, plants also require minerals. Although only a very small quantity of a plant comes from mineral substances in the soil this small proportion can be vital to growth. At least 16 elements are required in plant growth. Air and water supply carbon, hydrogen and oxygen. Nitrogen, potassium, calcium and phosphorus are required in considerable quantities, and plants obtain them via their roots. Magnesium, sulphur, manganese, boron, iron, zinc, copper, molybdenum and chlorine are required in very small amounts only. There is rarely any need to consider adding these to soil.

Figure 23 illustrates the nutrient cycle, or rather cycles, from a human centred point of view.

THE IMPORTANCE OF TREES

THE WATER CYCLE

Pharoah Akhnaten in a poem refers to 'lands whose Nile is in the sky'. The explanation of this strange phrase is that while most Egyptians of that period had never seen rain their armies had conquered many lands where it was common. Adequate rain is not found everywhere, nor can any supply of the most essential of all nutrients be taken for granted.

Water evaporates over the sea. Some of the resulting clouds drift towards the land, are forced upwards by high land masses, so cooling the clouds and precipitating rain. The resulting streams form rivers and return the water to the sea to complete the cycle. The cooling effect produced by the transpiration of forest trees can also produce precipitation of water as rain, so a region covered by forests can have the same influence on precipitating rain as elevated land masses.

FIGURE 24: THE WATER CYCLE

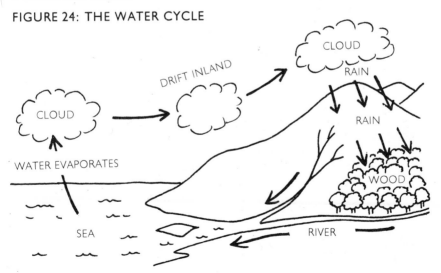

Trees also protect soil from desiccating winds and break the force of torrential rain, so reducing its erosion effects on the soil. Forests also retain moisture and hence life, and the effects of both floods and droughts are greatly mitigated by forests. Forests constitute a highly stable ecosystem within which the elements essential to life co-exist in dynamic equilibrium. Their present rapid destruction is a calamity and a menace to future generations. This applies especially to tropical forests whose destruction so frequently results in deserts. The destruction of forests has been going on for 5,000 years. The hills of Lebanon were famous for their trees, especially cedars, for thousands of years. Mount Lebanon is referred to in the Epic of Gilgamesh (before 2000 BC). The Pharoahs imported these cedars, King Solomon used them for his temple, and Alexander the Great used Lebanon timber to construct his Euphrates fleet. By the time of the Roman occupation of this region they had mainly gone. Today the hills are bare desert or scrub, apart from twelve or so preserved groves.

One third of the world's trees are in the Amazon's 5 million square kilometres of rain forest; by photosynthesis they supply nearly half the world's oxygen. But 40% of these forests have disappeared in the last century and at the present rate of destruction there will be little left by the year 2000. The rain forests of south east Asia are also being rapidly cut down. Photosynthesis in tropical forest trees proceeds at about ten times the rate of that in temperate climate trees which means they are much more effective in keeping constant the small proportion (0.03%) of carbon dioxide in the atmosphere. If this were to increase too much it could produce a 'greenhouse effect' and so lead to a general rise in temperature over the whole globe, with disastrous results (like the melting of the polar ice and the resulting raising of the ocean level world wide). An equal decrease in the oxygen level would be much less significant as there is 700 times as much oxygen as carbon dioxide in the atmosphere.

FIGURE 25: TIMBER USE WORLDWIDE

	Fuel 47%		Buildings, furniture etc. 43%	paper 10%

DESTRUCTION OF TROPICAL FORESTS AND DESERTIFICATION

Forests now cover about 20% of the earth's land surface. Tropical forests cover about 10%, some 900 million hectares (58% in South America, 19% in Africa, 22% in Asia and Oceania). A report in 1980, prepared for Jimmy Carter (*The Global 2000 Report to the President*) vividly described their past and forecast decline. 'Twenty two years ago forests covered one-fourth of the world's land surface. Now forests cover one-fifth. Twenty two years from now in the year 2000 forests are expected to have reduced to one-sixth of the land area. The world's forests are likely to stabilise at about one-seventh of the world's land area around the year 2030'.

Such declines are frequently irreversible. The decline has and will be almost all in the tropical forests; the area of temperate forest is not declining and is even increasing in some areas, but conifers have, as in the UK, replaced native broad leaved woodland with great ecological loss (a rich natural habitat is replaced by a very poor one).

Tropical forests are extremely old and constitute very stable ecosystems when undisturbed by 'civilised' humans. They are the home of a much greater diversity of flora and fauna than is found in temperate forests or elsewhere, and are also the home of native people with various lifestyles, who have lived in accord and understanding with their environment for centuries. Although undisturbed tropical forests form extremely stable ecosystems, these systems are very fragile when attacked, and tropical forests have been described as 'deserts covered by trees'. The rapid and **accelerating** decline of these forests could prove **as great a threat** to future life on earth as the possible nuclear holocaust.

FIGURE 26: EXPANDING DESERTS AND DECLINING FORESTS

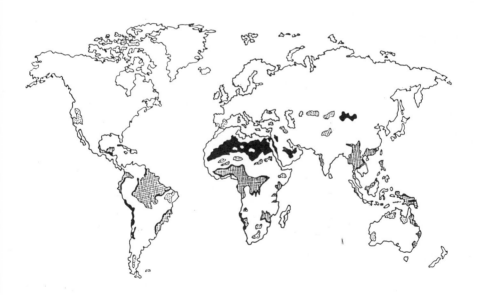

◆ Hyper arid areas (extreme desert) – 6% of the earth's ice-free land area

∴ Very high risk area – 3% of ice-free land area (semi desert)

▦ Tropical forests; dark areas here represent zones of forest undergoing rapid depletion; few forest areas (except inaccessible parts of western Amazonia and much of the Zaire Basin) are immune.

Gaia Atlas

Richard St. Barbe Baker used to say **'when trees go deserts come'**. He formed the 'Men of the Trees' organization in Kenya in 1922, and this world wide organisation has planted millions of trees around the world. In his book *Sahara Conquest* he described ways in which the Sahara could be reclaimed. Reclaimed because for 3,000 years or so (5500 to 2500 BC) forests flourished where the desert now is and wild game life abounded. After about 2500 BC primitive agriculture began. During the last 1,000 years great empires flourished in what is now the Sahel. Their existence implies an adequate supply of food and wood at this period. .

Forests are destroyed for timber, for firewood, for cultivation, and even recently by fire to form ranches for meat production and export. As soon as the protective cover of trees is removed the soil is exposed to erosion. It cracks in the hot sun and torrential rains wash it away. Remaining trees are undermined, low lying land is flooded, and growing crops destroyed. In a few years the habitat of a deforested area can be destroyed. In the tropics this process can be very rapid and even in areas where land can be successfully cultivated for a while, the soil can quickly deteriorate to the state where it has no further value.

Every month an area the size of Wales is felled. The FAO estimate that more than 11,137 thousand hectares of forest world wide are cleared each year to make way for agriculture and every year 253,820 thousand hectares (the area of England and Scotland combined) of once fertile land declines to the point where it will yield nothing. It is not possible to give any adequate account of this subject within the scope of this book but there are other matters which should at least be mentioned.

Native forest people have been the victims of genocide in the last few decades. Many thousands have been killed to make way for mines, ranches and roads. In the Matto Grosso, smallpox, influenza, and tuberculosis were deliberately introduced to reduce the numbers of native tribes. They have been bombed, and poisoned with arsenic added to their food. Government soldiers in Paraguay have hunted tribes people and shot them to clear areas wanted by business interests. In South America some two million Indians have 'disappeared' in Brazil alone. Native forest people did not produce population explosions.

During the last few decades multinational firms from Europe, North America and Japan have moved into tropical rainforest areas, to get quick profits from logging plantation forestry, ranching and mining. About 50 large USA based firms are so involved, with a somewhat smaller number of Japanese transnationals and firms based in Britain and European countries. Of course avaricious quick profits leave behind devastation. One of the worst of these is the destruction by fire to produce ranches for meat production. Many big agri-business barons are involved including well known names not usually associated with food. 'The largest ranch yet attempted, some 181,470 hectares, belongs to the German car manufacturer, Volkswagen. The pall of smoke created when the forest was burned to create pasture was visible by satellite picture, generating stern censure and a fine from the Brazilian government.' (*The Death of Trees* Nigel Dudley) .

Of course meat is a cash crop. 'In Costa Rica where vast forest areas were cleared to grow beef, production increased by 92% during the 1960s but home consumption fell by 26% in the same period, the rest being sold abroad, mainly in the USA.' (*The Death of Trees*).

The position in temperate forest regions is a quite different matter. Our downs and moors are not deserts only land partly ruined. Britain has fortunately an adequate rainfall and one spread over all seasons, but it has only some 7% or 8% of its land wooded whereas Sweden has about 64%. In Europe only Iceland and Ireland have less. The problem in Britain (and in Europe) is that conifer plantations have replaced natural woodlands. The natural forests that do remain in Britain are often slowly degenerating. In the Snowdonia National Park over 90% of the woodlands are failing to regenerate because sheep are eating the young saplings and preventing regrowth. Highlands should be covered by native trees not sheep.

A very interesting and much fuller account of these matters is given in *The Death of Trees* (SEE booklist).

HOW MUCH FOOD FROM A HECTARE?

Relative energy and protein yields per hectare are not necessarily those per kilogram of the food in question. For example wheat and peas have a higher protein content per kilogram than potatoes but a crop of peas (32.3 kg/hectare) gives less than half the protein per hectare of potatoes (67.9 kg/hectare) because the potato yield per hectare is much higher than that of peas.

Table 12 illustrates this point. While the data are from various sources and not precise they do give a good general indication.

TABLE 12: PROTEIN AND ENERGY YIELDS

Product harvested	Protein kg/hectare/year	Energy M cal/hectare/year
Leaf protein	327.7	1,312
Cabbage (edible)	180.3	3,932
Potato (edible tuber)	67.9	2,459
Barley grain (UK)	60.6	2,295
Milk (cow)	56.5	409
Chicken (edible broiler)	18.9	180
Eggs	13.0	188
Beef (edible meat, mainly barley fed)	9.4	180
Pig (edible meat)	8.3	309
Lamb (edible meat, UK & Eire)	3.7–7.9	203–506
Beef (edible meat, mainly grass fed)	4.4	300

Various sources

PROTEIN AND ENERGY EFFICIENCY

If the protein we get from eating an animal is only one-tenth of the protein fed to the animal, the efficiency of protein production is 10%; if the energy obtained from eating an animal product is one-fifth of the energy in the feed supplied to an animal the energy efficiency is one-fifth or 20%. A low efficiency means that most of the protein or energy fed to the animal is wasted.

FIGURE 27: ANIMAL PROTEIN AND ENERGY YIELDS

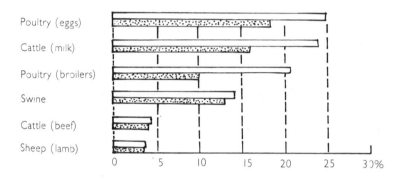

☐ Protein yield from the product as a percentage of the protein supplied as feed to the livestock.

▨ Energy obtained from the product as a percentage of the energy supplied as feed to the livestock.

This diagram shows how inefficient animal produce is as a way of obtaining protein and energy.

Scientific American September 1976

THE CHANGING FACE OF AGRICULTURE

Agriculture in most developed world countries developed gradually over centuries and was adapted to suit the climate, means, circumstances and requirements. (It did also in Third World countries but colonialism harmed it there.) In recent decades as a result of green revolution techniques and a combination of private enterprise and public subsidies, like the CAP in Europe, it has been 'too successful by half' and produced the notorious lakes and mountains of surplus products.

The green revolution has, on the whole, been disastrous for the world's poor. It has succeeded in producing more food in many countries but at the cost of destroying traditional methods which were well adapted to climate and other local conditions, and also at the cost of eliminating small farmers who, all too often, cannot afford new seeds, fertilizers and more irrigation all together. It has thus concentrated land ownership in the hands of a few. For example in North East Brazil 9% of landowners now possess over 80% of the land and many previous owners and tenant farmers now seek work. Mechanisation is making their position worse. As in other Third World countries, the many who relied on the land for sustenance and employment can no longer do so. The food they grew has in effect been taken from them. There is nothing so ruthless and anti-social as a free market economy except war and some dictatorships.

In Britain the richest 9% of the population own 84% of the land, and as in poor countries, new farming techniques have tended to reduce the number of land holdings, but as less than 3% of the work force work directly on the land and there is a welfare state, this in itself does not directly produce dire poverty and want.

As in eighteenth and nineteenth century Britain, after the theft of the land enclosures, there is a drift in the Third World to the cities. They have expanded at a fantastic rate. Unlike 18th and 19th century Britain, most Third World countries have huge debts on which crippling interest has to be paid which means that economics takes precedence over ecology — today's want over tomorrow's need. In short, cash crops are grown, and the debts paid, when possible; the poor can starve and the land deteriorate.

Examples of the effect of cash crops and soil deterioration have been given in other sections. Meat is a most costly cash crop as far as the poor of the developing countries are concerned. In the Kalahari desert of Botswana, one of the world's last natural places, large areas of land have been fenced in to prevent the spread of foot and mouth disease among the enclosed cattle, a special semi-wild hybrid animal suited to these conditions. The 3,000 kilometres of fences have however produced a heavy death toll of the native wildebeest. In 1983 at least 50,000 wildebeest died of thirst because the steel fences prevented their migration to sources of water. The industry produces 500,000 tonnes per day of corned beef and pet food and it is worth $100 million a year — but what will the final cost be in ecological damage?

PESTICIDES

All pesticides used should later disintegrate into harmless products and never be persistent. DDT is an example of a persistent insecticide that should not have been used. It is still present in nature and affecting animal health and behaviour — causing a mother seal to kill her own cubs, for example. Rachel Carson's book *Silent Spring* is a classic on the devastation produced by careless and excessive use of pesticides. There is a clear need for stricter government control of pesticides.

Other forms of pollution can also have harmful effects on plants and animals; for example the anti-skid salt spread on roads kills trees when the salt grit is left in heaps near them; it is also destructive of life when it gets into streams and rivers.

LAND DISTRIBUTION AND USE

The richest 1% of Britain's population owns 52% of all land, while the poorest 80% own 7.8% of the land between them. Land is 28.5% of the total wealth. (SEE figure 28)

FIGURE 28: OWNERSHIP OF LAND IN BRITAIN

The numbers give the area
in million hectares

Each dot represents 1% of the population (563,000).

The area of the circle represents the total land area (24.1 million hectares).

2.0

2.0

2.4

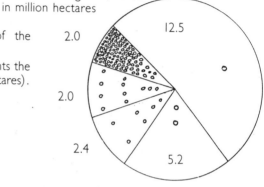

12.5

5.2

SERA *New Ground*
Autumn 1985

TABLE 15: LAND OWNERSHIP AND WEALTH

Population group	Share of all wealth	Share of total land	Average land per person
Richest 1%	17%	52%	22 hectares
Next richest 2%	17.5%	21.7%	4.6 hectares
Next richest 6%	12%	10.4%	0.73 hectares
Next richest 11%	15.8%	8.1%	0.32 hectares
Poorest 80%	37.7%	7.8%	0.04 hectares

SERA *New Ground*
Autumn 1985

In England and Wales about two-thirds of land holdings are under 40 hectares and occupy one-tenth of the land area; the remaining one-third occupies nine-tenths of the total land area. The distribution in the rest of Europe is more even, but as FAO figures show, it is even more uneven in the Third World where on average 2.5% of landowners with holdings over 200 hectares control three-quarters of all land, with the top 0.23% controlling over half.

The use of land in Britain is shown in figure 29. About 75% of all arable land is devoted to animal upkeep, and as animals have protein and calorie efficiencies well below 20% this is very wasteful of resources. It requires heavy inputs of fertilizers.

FIGURE 29: LAND USE IN BRITAIN

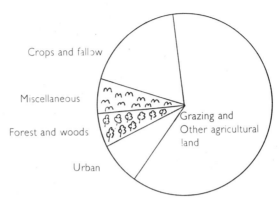

Crops and fallow

Miscellaneous

Forest and woods

Urban

Grazing and Other agricultural land

Economic Development Council statistics

In terms of consumption people are not all that much of a burden on this planet. Their domestic animals are several times more so. There are at any time about three million tonnes of human beings in Britain and about nine million tonnes of animals (cattle, sheep, pigs and poultry, etc.). The animals have a much shorter lifespan than the humans (broiler fowl live only seven weeks) and so have a much higher rate of consumption.

FIGURE 30: POPULATION OF UK

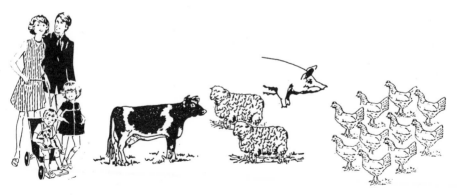

3 millon tonnes of humans, 9 million tonnes of animals

56 million humans, 14 million cattle, 28 million sheep, 8 million pigs, 142 million poultry

4 humans to: 1 cow or beef beast + 2 sheep + 0.6 pig + 10 poultry

FIGURE 31: LAND USE IN THE UK per average family

Total land 24.1 million hectares; agricultural land 19.15 million hectares

FOR FOUR PEOPLE:

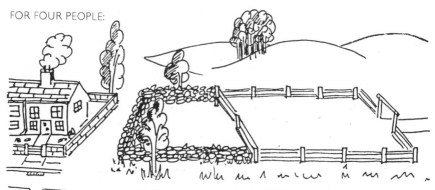

Typical semi on 400 sq. m. | 3,240 sq. m to grow food direct for people. | 10,520 sq. m to provide food for animals plus land abroad for further fodder.

We feed most of our home grown grain to animals and import some bread wheat and other animal feeding stuffs. Exports are required to pay for this — involving more factories, more energy used, less garden space for houses, allotments etc. Some 75% or 80% of our land is devoted, directly and indirectly, to animal products. On the other hand, as NEDC agriculture figures show, meat and animal products are about two-thirds, in cash terms, of the agricultural industry's output. Agriculture employs about 2% to 3% of the total national manpower and contributes about the same to the Gross Domestic Product.

AGRICULTURE AND EMPLOYMENT

For many thousands of years, since the first agricultural revolution, most people were employed directly in agriculture. This is still the case in many developing countries. The contemporary position (1976) is illustrated in figure 32.

FIGURE 32: LABOUR FORCE IN AGRICULTURE

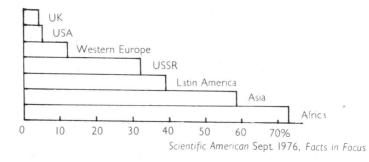

Scientific American Sept. 1976, Facts in Focus

In Britain in 1900 there were one million horses eating one-third of the annual agricultural output. In 1965, there were only 2,000 working horses left. In 1935 there were about 20,000 tractors; in 1974 there were 500,000.

In 1820 the USA employed over 70% of its labour force on the land — now it is about 5%. During the period 1910 to 1970 the absolute output of farms in the USA approximately doubled, with a declining labour force. In the UK 2.5% to 3% of the labour force produces over half the indigenous food consumed and could easily produce all with a modified diet. If one were to grow most of the average family's food the equivalent of five or six weeks full-time labour per annum could suffice. For this change from the drudgery of earlier times credit must go to modern technology, including 'artificial' fertilizers, improved plant strains, pesticides, machinery, etc., even if some of these are overdone. Importing any of our indigenous food is expensive and unnecessary, as is also the Common Agricultural Policy.

WHAT IS THE POSITION REGARDING ALLOTMENTS?

Allotments go back to the Middle Ages. In the reign of Elizabeth I they were made to compensate labourers for the loss of common land; till the nineteenth century they generally came from private benefactors. There was an Allotments Act in 1887 compelling allotment authorities to provide allotments where demand was known to exist. By 1985 there were 450,000 allotments, usually under 1,000 square metres. The demand for allotments went up during both World Wars and dropped afterwards — it is now again high and likely to remain so.

> In 1969 there were 7,000 waiting applicants; 560,625 allotments of area 24,370 hectares or 0.1% of total land area.
> In 1977 there were 120,000 waiting applicants; 498,605 allotments of area 20,180 hectares or 0.08% of total land area.
>
> *Economic Growth*

There is much derelict and despoiled land in Britain. Official estimates give about 44,520 hectares — unofficial estimates about ten times as much. Vacant land in London has been estimated at 3,100 hectares.

Increased availability of allotments is most desirable on social and economic grounds as high food prices and high unemployment are likely to remain.

WHAT ABOUT FACTORY FARMING?

Between 1945 and 1976 animal production in the UK expanded dramatically.

Cattle:	8.5 million to 14 million
Sheep:	19 million to 28 million
Pigs:	2 million to 8 million
Poultry:	4 million to 142 million

This expansion was made possible by factory farming, an inhumane business where animals are kept in extremely cramped conditions. It has its opponents but as animal products and meat produce two-thirds of the profits from farming it has increased and prospered. Much of it is owned by big business firms and multinationals, such as Spillers French.

Factory farming

1)   is wasteful of resources;

2)   has a dehumanising effect on its workers;

3)   is a health hazard, e.g. drug resistant bacteria can be produced in animals by extensive use of antibiotics, build-up of accumulative poisons (e.g. arsenic — a growth promoter — hormones, etc.);

4)   leads to deteriorating food values e.g. eggs with reduced B12 and folic acid content;

5)   gives rise to serious effluent problems — fouling of waterways etc.;

6)   is an environmental nuisance and an eyesore, produces indescribable stenches which have led to court actions.

It has nevertheless received favourable treatment from the authorities — exemption from rates, grants for buildings, ease or exemption from planning permission, compensation for loss of stock through diseases, etc. Its purpose is increased profits and reduced labour costs. It is **big** business.

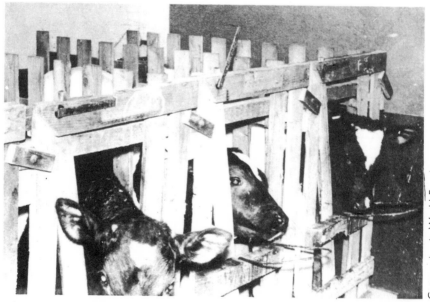

Compassion in World Farming

Factory farming is quite unacceptable for both ecological and compassionate reasons. It is a typical example of government neglect and evasion of a difficult problem or moral dilemma. A committee of enquiry, chaired by Professor Roger Bramwell, reported in 1965. Dealing with calves, for example, it laid down five freedoms for their treatment and recommended their legal enforcement. No action was taken till 1967 when the Agriculture (Miscellaneous Provisions) Bill was introduced; it became law in 1968. It enabled the Minister to make regulations, which he did not do, and to issue Codes of Practice, which became voluntary codes and ineffectual. There were debates in both Houses in October 1976. The system was generally condemned, but had its defenders, for example William Ross, then Secretary of State for Scotland: 'turning round may not be advisable from the point of view of the animal' and David Ensor, declaring an interest in the poultry industry: 'I doubt if there are many children in this country who live under such comfortable circumstances as these birds do . . .' Those who have seen intensive poultry houses or photographs thereoff will find this last statement extraordinary. The recommendations have been watered down to the point of virtual rejection.

In November 1969 the Swann Committee gave its report on the dangers of the continuous use of hormones and antibiotics in factory farming in building up drug resistant bacteria. Harmless resistant bacteria are capable of transmitting drug resistance to pathogenic bacteria and so are a potential health hazard to those who eat the produce of factory farms, or even come into contact with it. The danger lies in the fact that if the person caught a germ, usually treated with the antibiotic involved, the antibiotic would probably prove ineffectual.

Factory farming only comes about because of the very high consumption of meat and animal products in the rich world, the greed of producers and their desire for large profits and so to employ as few workers as possible.

THE 'MUCK AND MAGIC' FALLACY

This is the notion that animals somehow enrich the soil by just feeding on its produce and returning the dung thereto. They can only return some of the nutrients they have taken from it. Any crop, vegetable or animal, must subtract something from the soil. Of course where animals are fed on imported food, fodder, this is no longer true. There is then a case of **imported fertility** — a very expensive way of doing it; it is also a matter of robbing Peter's soil to enrich Paul's. While so-called 'artificial' manures can be overdone and lack the carbon-containing material of natural wastes, all crops, animal or vegetable, take nutrient elements from the soil (except legumes in the case of nitrogen). The ecological cycle is not complete unless human sewage is treated and recycled. 'Artificial' or chemical fertilizers are at present essential to sustained production though full use should and is made of all waste products. If domestic food animals did not consume so much of the vegetable food produced and in effect occupy so much of our land area for such a low return less chemical fertilizers would be required.

Humus is a most important factor in soil fertility. It affects soil structure, moisture holding properties and the pH value (acidity or alkalinity) of a soil; the latter affects the nutrient exchange between soil and plant — so adding peat to a clay soil, for example, can produce an increase in fertility far beyond the simple carbon addition involved.

For a fuller discussion of these matters and the subject of organic cultivation (a method of farming and gardening which avoids all chemical fertilizers and pesticides by making the fullest use of organic wastes and composts) see booklist and addresses at the end of this book.

SMALL MIXED FARMS

Small mixed farms are sometimes put forward as panaceas for our agricultural ills. While small holdings are often more efficient than larger ones, a small farm with animals is all too likely to develop into one producing meat and dairy produce only, crops being grown just to feed the animals. The majority of our farms support animals, as MAFF statistics show (SEE Land distribution and use). What is really wrong with our agriculture is that too much of our food resources are diverted to supporting animals, whose efficiency as food converters is low. Horticulture needs to increase and animal farming to decrease.

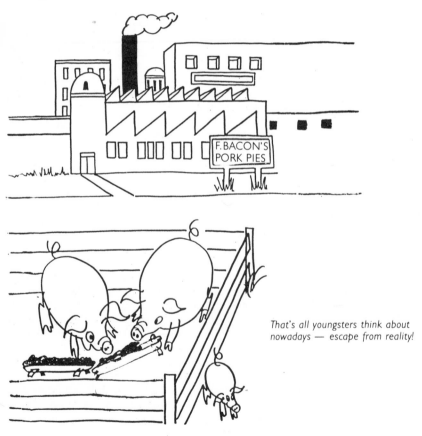

That's all youngsters think about nowadays — escape from reality!

7 RESUME AND CONCLUSION

THE ENIGMA

The main theme of this book is the problem of starvation and malnutrition in a world where food is produced to excess, and in fact deliberately destroyed in quantities more than enough to meet any want had there been the will to so use it (the logistics involved would have been easily solved had 'defence' been involved). This is the enigma or, as Nigel Twose expresses it in *Cultivating Hunger*: 'What kind of a world is it that seeks a solution to its sophisticated problems of high finance by taking away food from the poor?' The answer is all too obvious **to those who wish to see it** — in short a world of ruthless exploitation.

IMPLICATIONS OF POPULATION GROWTH

Of course the problem of poverty (the cause of want and inevitable result of insatiable greed) is greatly aggravated by rapid population increase. When a poor country has a 4% per annum rate of population increase, which means a doubling period of about 17½ years, the situation is not helped by a visiting prominent world religious leader, preaching 'Humanae Vitae' and condemning 'Liberation Theology', or by the inhabitants of such countries being too poor to buy contraceptives. One result of such population explosions, in poor countries, is the need for cash crops to pay interest on foreign loans, which in turn results in the poorest people in increasing numbers trying to subsist on marginal land, and that in its turn results in famine and disaster. Increasing over-population, at present, is due to increasing life span as well as to high birth rate; high birth rate is usually greatest in the very poor countries. There are however many countries where a population policy is necessary and some (as in China) where compulsory family size limitation is justified for the common good.

It is over simplistic to attribute starvation in the Third World simply to population increase. In Africa and South America where there is most unused land available (SEE What population could the land feed?) there is also most malnutrition and starvation. People are even found starving on or near land which they could use to grow food, as in the case of Senegal (SEE Introduction). Those who could cultivate the land to grow their own food can't, while those who own the land will not allow it to be used except for profit.

However over-population does diminish human freedom and it leads to the loss of the remaining wilderness — to which the wisest have from earliest times resorted to meditate and regain sanity. But even there the domestic animal over-population is as important (as in the case of meat production in the Kalahari Desert in Botswana — SEE The changing face of agriculture).

Exploitation is the main cause of starvation and malnutrition. The poor in the poor countries are exploited by their own rich (and also by intruders from richer countries), while the richer over-developed countries exploit the poorer ones. Eco-catastrophe and so-called 'Acts of God' are at most contributory factors. If there were more compassion and less senseless greed in the world mass starvation would not occur; and neither also would the exploitation of animals and the environment.

ECOLOGICAL BLUNDERS AND DETERIORATION

A striking example of an ecological blunder and disregard of traditional lifestyles was given in an article in *Malawi News*(3rd October 1969). All over the East Bank of the Lower River, twenty years earlier, a four metre high thatch grass (parrhenia) grew. Women going to draw water at the streams had someone walk in front to find or make a path for them. Cultivated patches of maize had an emerald green grass called msonthi growing among them which helped to keep them wet. Rice patches were also grown. The ground was always damp and if rivers flooded in rainy periods the thick vegetation trapped the silt. An early flowering sorghum (gugu) grew wild and provided a food reserve between one crop and the next. The rains came regularly when expected. Then along came the 'improvers' (forestry officials in uniform). They had all the thatch grass removed and burnt for several years. The final result was the land became hard baked in dry spells and silt was washed away in rainy periods. It was a total catastrophe. The hills once covered by trees were by then only sparsely clad.

This is a special case, but typical of what is happening in African and Third World countries. The destruction of tropical forests is one of the largest in scale and potential consequences. Acid rain, chemical pollution of rivers and the North Sea, and the ever-increasing accumulation of long-life radioactive waste from nuclear reactors are others. Further examples of ecological deterioration have been described (SEE Destruction of tropical forests and desertification).

ANIMAL EXPLOITATION

This subject has been discussed in 'Factory Farming' and 'The Vegan Diet'. The national press in 1984 carried the story of a two year old cow, Blackie. She was sent to market with her first-born calf. They were sold to separate farmers, seven miles apart. Next morning the farmer who had bought the calf was surprised to find it had acquired a mother. Blackie had jumped a gate and managed the long trek through the dark. The farmer's wife said 'We will buy her. They will stay together. I am a mother myself and can imagine what she felt like'. (*What happens to the cow and calf* Movement for Compassionate Living). This is an unusual case. The common sequel to separation is tragic and pathetic.

Milk and its products are not even healthy foods. Milk can carry serious infections, such as salmonellosis, brucellosis, tuberculosis and campylobacter. Intolerance to it can cause eczema, asthma, tonsillitis and internal disturbances especially in children. If it were not so usual the continuous consumption throughout its whole life of the infant food of another animal (i.e. cow's milk) and products made therefrom would be seen as absurd as it in fact is.

HUMAN EXPLOITATION

Those who treat animals as mere machines find it easy to treat human beings as just other animals. For example, Dan Ellerman of the US National Security Council said in 1974 '. . . to give food aid to countries just because people are starving is a pretty weak reason'. Senator Hubert Humphrey, later Vice President, with some reputation for liberalism, said in 1957 'I have heard . . . that people may become dependent on us for food. I know that is not supposed to be good news. To me, that was good news, because before people can do anything else they have got to eat. And if you are looking for a way to get people to lean on you and be dependent on you in terms of co-operation with you, it seems to me that food dependence would be terrific'. The technique of animal training applied to human beings! But a view not unique; a CIA Research Report expresses a similar view. Lust for power is a most pernicious form of greed; it is a much more potent 'source of evil' than mere 'love of money' (even if the latter sometimes leads to the former).

One should remember also the ever-growing power of big business and the multinationals (power without responsibility); it is a potential threat to human freedom, democracy, and humane values. They are already more wealthy than some states, and if nothing is done, could in future take over national states. One has already disposed of an elected government in Chile. World wide they may well be exerting a much greater power than most people would imagine.

Exploitation of animals in today's world all too often means human exploitation also. Examples of this have been given but here are two more from *Food First*:

In Mexico more basic grains are consumed by livestock than by the country's peasants.

Brazil and Paraguay have been rapidly expanding soya bean acreage (largely through foreign investment); yet almost all of this protein rich food is for export to fatten livestock.

These are three countries with much poverty, hunger and malnutrition.

'What I want to see above all else is that this country remains a country where someone can always get rich. That's the thing we have and that must be preserved.'

Ronald Reagan

THE ROLE OF FALSE VALUES

Humans are theorizing and conceptualizing animals which is why they have become increasingly able to control their environment, but lack self control. And also why, unless unusually well informed and thoughtful, they are easily impressed by, dominated by, and even intoxicated by, ideas — from irrational dogmas to advertisers' pressures. Also why a wealth-controlled mass media and the yellow press are able to effect a consensus of opinion and greatly influence what people eat, drink, wear and so on. Acquisitive greed and gainful competition are represented as the only reliable incentives and social co-operation as impractical idealism — greed as the cardinal virtue and the Economy as God.

Neocolonialism, the system of unfair exchange which means over half the world's population supply the rich nations with necessary raw materials at declining returns, because they have incurred ever-increasing debts, is mainly ignored, as is also the complete disregard for human rights when it suits the powerful rich nations. A particularly disgraceful example of such occurred when Britain evicted the 1,800 inhabitants of Diego Garcia (1965–1973) from their island homes, where they had lived for centuries, to make way for a USA naval base. They were deposited destitute on Mauritius (although they were then British citizens — but black). Their treatment was a complete disgrace to Britain and discreditable to the USA and Mauritius. It was kept dark for years. It forms a stark contrast to the Falklands, where we must have spent some £5 million per family. There were about 1,800 inhabitants in each case.

Poverty is created by greed. A greed motivated society will inevitably produce want and misery somewhere — and eventually its own destruction.

AN ECOLOGICAL ANSWER

There is a wide gulf between the present exploitative economics and the ecological 'green' outlook, between profit first and the common interest. This was discussed in 'Ecology and Conventional Economics'. Unfortunately the outlook that disfigured the face of Britain in the nineteenth century and most of this one, and did much greater harm elsewhere, still prevails and we are throwing away much of the welfare of future generations for the senseless lust for gain of a few today.

The green view puts co-operation before competition, sufficiency before lust for gain, social service before money making, conserving essential non-renewable resources before their squandering for today's greed.

A vegetarian or vegan diet is sound ecology. It takes five or more times (informed estimates vary) as much land to feed a meat eater as it does a vegan. But as in the UK meat, poultry and dairy products form two-thirds of the farmers' income and employ two-thirds of the labour involved, economic profitability, or market economics, is in favour of their maintenance, even if they take up most of the food subsidies. There are many better uses for land than producing subsidized surplus food.

Evidence of a recent poll suggests that millions of people are reducing their meat consumption and many are becoming vegetarians. It is an understandable reaction to a growing recognition of the cruelty and wastefulness of animal farming and the demands our meat centred diet makes on the Third World. Others, aware of the cruelty and demand on resources of milk and dairy production, would carry the protest still further by going entirely vegan. Without food animals even the over populated UK could feed far more than its present population and have land over for other purposes.

We grow twice as much food on this planet each year as is necessary to give anyone an adequate diet, but we are obsessed with animal protein. The consumption of meat is not just a question of cruelty to animals, but of cruelty to people.

Sir Bernard Wetherall, Speaker of the House of Commons

REFERENCES AND SOURCES OF INFORMATION

The author has used a great many different sources in writing this book. Many are given in the text, but the main references for each section are listed below. Full bibliographical details are given in the booklist.

The following sources were extensively used for statistical information.

Facts in Focus
UK Annual Abstract of Statistics
United Nations Statistical Yearbook
United Nations Demographic Yearbook
The New State of the World Atlas M Kidron and R Segal
Gaia Atlas of Planet Management Norman Myers

I: Introduction
North–South and Common Crisis Brandt Commission
Farming in the Clouds Richard Body
The Seventh Enemy Ronald Higgins

2: The World Food Problem
The State of Food and Agriculture FAO
Scientific American September 1976
North–South and Common Crisis Brandt Commission
Population Roland Pressat
Vegetarian Society and Vegan Society publications

3: Growth, Economics and Neocolonialism
North–South and Common Crisis Brandt Commission
Campaign against the Arms Trade publications
Unnatural Disaster, Oxfam News and other publications Oxfam
The Tea Trade and Spur World Development Movement
Agscene Compassion in World Farming
Unilever Counter Information Services
How the Other Half Dies Susan George
The Baby Killer and The Baby Killer Scandal War on Want

4: The Political Background
North and South and Common Crisis Brandt Commission
Creation of World Poverty Teresa Hayter
Aid, Rhetoric and Reality Teresa Hayter and Catharine Watson
Aid is Not Enough Independent Group on British Aid
Hungry for Change newsletter Oxfam
The Triumph and the Shame and Farming in the Clouds Richard Body
World Development Movement publications

5: Nutrition, Fact and Fancy
Scientific American September 1976
Diet for a Small Planet Frances Moore Lappe
Outline of Vegetarian Nutrition W.S. James
Vegan Nutrition Frey Ellis and T. Saunders
Vegan Compost and B12 Kathleen Jannaway
National Food Surveys Ministry of Agriculture, Food and Fisheries
The Law and the Loaf K. Barlow
Vegan Society publications

6: Food, Ecology and Agriculture
The Death of Trees Nigel Dudley
Economic Growth Pete Riley
Compassion in World Farming publications
Vegan Society publications

BOOKLIST

This list includes details of the books to which the author refers in the text, and which he used in writing *Food: Need, Greed and Myopia.* It is not a comprehensive list of books on world food issues but gives suggestions for further reading. Many of the books listed will include bibliographies and reading lists. Not all the books are still in print; it should be possible to find those that are not in libraries.

General

Facts in Focus Central Statistical Office (Penguin) 255 pages
A book of UK statistics and a valuable source of reference on many topics.
UK Annual Abstract of Statistics (HMSO, annual)
Comprehensive statistics.
United Nations Statistical Yearbook (HMSO, annual)
An invaluable source of statistics.
United Nations Demographic Yearbook (annual)
Very detailed population statistics.
New State of the World Atlas M Kidron & R Segal (Pan 1984) 176 pages, 65 maps
Covers most contemporary aspects of poverty and exploitation. A valuable source of information.
Gaia Atlas of Planet Management edited by Norman Myers (Pan 1985) 272 pages
Text, maps and diagrams on aspects of global management. A valuable source of information even if it is not always sure if it rejects or accepts values of conventional market economics.
Population Roland Pressat (translated from French) (Pelican 1973) 152 pages
A most readable, thorough and valuable account of the subject.
The Economic History of World Population Carlo Ciopalla (Pelican 1962) 125 pages
Population R K Kelsall (Longmans 1967)
Deals with Britain only.

Aid, Trade and Development; Neocolonialism

Small is Beautiful: a study of economics as if people mattered E F Schumacher (Abacus 1974) 256 pages
A best seller which thoroughly deserved to be. Deals with the moral, psychological, social and ecological aspects of economics.
The Limits to Growth D Meadows et al (Pan 1972) 208 pages
The first report of the Club of Rome's project on the predicament of man.
Mankind at the Turning Point M Mesarovic and E Pestel (PE Dutton 1976) 223 pages
The second report of the Club of Rome. Food, ecological and population problems.

The Seventh Enemy: the human factor in the global crisis Ronald Higgins (Pan 1978) 286 pages
An interesting and readable account of the psychological and other aspects of the world situation.

North–South: a programme for survival Brandt Commission (Pan 1980) 308 pages
A report of the Independent Commission on International Development Issues under the chairmanship of Willy Brandt.

Common Crisis: North–South Co-operation for World Recovery (Pan Books 1983) 174 pages
The most recent report of the Independent Commission chaired by Willy Brandt.

Aid and the Third World: The North/South Divide Guy Arnold (Robert Royce 1985) 180 pages

The Creation of World Poverty: an alternative view to the Brandt Report Teresa Hayter (Pluto 1981) 128 pages
This is a most valuable book. It shows clearly how Third World poverty was created and is being intentionally and unintentionally sustained.

Poverty and Power Rachael Heatley (Zed Press 1979) 96 pages
A case for a political approach to development and its implications for action in the west. A very readable and informative book.

Aid, Rhetoric and Reality Teresa Hayter and Catharine Watson (Pluto 1985) 288 pages
The false nature of aid and the role of financial institutions in maintaining poverty.

Real Aid: a strategy for Britain Independent Group on British Aid (1982) 61 pages
Their first report.

Aid is Not Enough: Britain and the world's poor Independent Group on British Aid (1984) 60 pages
Their second report.
These two books are full critical accounts of how aid works in action, examined by a group of seven men all experienced in development work (chairman, Professor Charles Elliott). The second is the more critical. Distributed by Oxfam, Christian Aid, World Development Movement and the Overseas Development Institute.

Against the Grain: the dilemma of project food aid A Jackson and D Eade (Oxfam 1982) 132 pages

The Third World Tomorrow Paul Harrison (Penguin 1980) 384 pages
An interesting first hand report on how the Third World poor are co-operating to help themselves.

The Tea Trade John Tanner and Roger Jeffrey (World Development Movement 1980) 48 pages
The human results of economic exploitation involved in this important cash crop.

Unacceptable Faces of Tea: James Finlay of Glasgow Farouk Faisal and Roger Jeffrey (SEAD Campaigns 1983) 20 pages
The ruthless exploitation of the Glasgow based firm of James Finlay.

The Baby Killer War on Want
The Baby Killer Scandal Andrew Chetley (War on Want 1979) 208 pages
War on Want's investigations into the promotion and sale of powdered baby milks in the Third World.

Cultivating Hunger: an Oxfam study of food, power and poverty Nigel Twose (Oxfam 1985) 48 pages
Why the Poor Suffer Most — drought and the Sahel Public Affairs Unit (Oxfam 1984) 20 pages
An Unnatural Disaster — drought in North East Brazil Public Affairs Unit (Oxfam 1984) 16 pages
Lessons Unlearned — drought and famine in Ethiopia Public Affairs Unit (Oxfam 1984) 18 pages
These books have been referred to in the text; they are full of useful information.

Diego Garcia — A contrast to the Falklands (Minority Rights Group 1982)
One of over 70 such reports to date.

Unilever Counter Information Services 102 pages
One of a number of reports on multinationals

Under the Eagle Jenny Pearce (Latin American Bureau 1982) 295 pages
US intervention in Central America and the Caribbean.

Food and its production; Agriculture

Food and Agriculture *Scientific American* September 1976
The whole issue looked at aspects of agriculture, food production and nutrition.

The State of Food and Agriculture 1984 FAO (1985) 185 pages
Detailed statistics on world agriculture and food production.

How the Other Half Dies: the real reason for world hunger Susan George (Pelican 1976) 352 pages
A full account of the world nutrition problem.

Ill Fares the Land Susan George (Writers and Readers 1985) 128 pages

Food for Beginners Susan George and Nigel Paige (new ed. Unwin 1986) 176 pages

More Than We Can Chew: the crazy world of food farming Charlie Clutterbuck and Tim Lang (Pluto 1982) 120 pages

Food First Frances Moore Lappe and Joseph Collins (Abacus 1982) 416 pages
The rich are starving the poor for profit — this book shows how.

The Famine Business Colin Tudge (Penguin 1979)

Food, Poverty and Power Anne Buchanan (Spokesman 1983) 123 pages

Food Resources Conventional and Novel N W Pirie (Penguin 1969) 208 pages
The scientific side of agriculture and horticulture and future prospects.

The Triumph and the Shame Richard Body (Temple Smith 1982)
Farming in the Clouds Richard Body (Temple Smith 1984) 161 pages
These books show clearly the tragic absurdities of the CAP, its futile extravagance and waste of resources, the ecological damage resulting from its policies and its harmful effects on the Third World countries. They deal also with the disastrous effects of EEC membership on Britain's economy and its role in producing unemployment.

Can Britain Feed Itself? Kenneth Mellanby (Merlin Press 1977) 90 pages

Changing Food Habits in the UK Chris Wardle (Earth Resources Research 1977) 98 pages
Full of interesting information and statistics. It deals with the monopoly aspect of food matters. Very valuable to a serious student of food problems.
Economic Growth Pete Riley (Friends of the Earth 1979) 62 pages
A most useful book about allotments.
The Law and the Loaf Kenneth Barlow (Precision Press 1978) 70 pages
Our Daily Bread Richard James (Penguin 1973) 96 pages
An account of five centuries of exploitation and the resulting effect of malnutrition on the nation's health. Well illustrated and full of useful interesting information.

Nutrition

Diet for a Small Planet Frances Moore Lappe (Ballantine 1975) 412 pages
A best seller. Deals fully with the principles of complementary sources and other nutritional mattes as well as the world food position; many recipes (not vegan).
Recipes for a Small Planet Ellen B Ewald (Ballantine 1978) 412 pages
Continues the theme of Diet for a Small Planet *with many more recipes (not vegan)*
Food for a Future: the ecological priority of a humane diet Jon Wynne Tyson (Centaur Press 1979) 160 pages
This is a most readable book full of information, dietary data, quotations etc.
E for Additives Maurice Hanssen (Thorsons 1984) 223 pages
A complete guide to the E numbers found on the lists of ingredients. Unfortunately it does not show if their origin is vegetable, mineral or animal.
The 1985-86 International Vegetarian Handbook Vegetarian Society (Thorsons 1985) 358 pages
Much useful information of interest to vegetarians and vegans including E numbers and the origins of the substances used.
Outline of Vegetarian Nutrition W S James (Vegetarian Society 1977) 12 pages
Vegetarian Nutrition Jack W Lucas (Vegetarian Society 1980) 136 pages
Valuable for anyone who wants to explore nutrition in greater depth.

Veganism

Vegan Nutrition Frey Ellis and T Saunders (Vegan Society 1985) 24 pages
Adequate information for most readers.
Why Vegan? Kath Clements (Heretic Books, GMP Publishers Ltd) 96 pages
A simple and effective statement of the vegan case. A good read.
First Hand, First Rate Kathleen Jannaway (Vegan Society 1976) 24 pages
60 simple recipes and ideas for economic living on largely home-produced food. Excellent value.
Vegan Cookery Eva Batt (Thorsons 1985) 144 pages
Practical advice and nourishing vegan recipes.
Vegan Cooking Leah Leneman (Thorsons 1982) 128 pages
Advice and appetising nourishing vegan recipes.

Vegan Compost and Vitamin B12 Kathleen Jannaway

Sustaining and Sustainable Kathleen Jannaway (Movement for Compassionate Living) 22 pages
The case for self-reliant living free from misuse of people (especially in the Third World), of animals, and of the environment. With menus, recipes and nutritional information.

Jack Sanderson, Man for a Future (Movement for Compassionate Living) 65 pages
Extracts from the writings of Jack Sanderson from The Vegan *(1958-83)*

New Whole Ways (Movement for Compassionate Living)
Imaginative whole food vegan recipes using only ingredients that could be home grown.

Factory Farming

Animal Machines Ruth Harrison (Vincent Stuart 1964)
A classic book on factory farming.

Animals, Man and Morals edited by Stanley Godlovitch (Gollanz 1976) 288 pages
Various aspects of the human treatment of animals.

The Animal Liberation Movement Peter Singer (Old Hammond Press)

Factory Farming Ruth Harrison

Factory Farming edited by J R Bellerby (British Association for the Advancement of Science 1970) 124 pages
Various papers on the subject, including the efficiency of animals as protein converters.

Assault and Battery: what factory farming means for humans and animals Mark Gold (Pluto 1983) 172 pages

Alternatives to Factory Farming: An Economic Appraisal Paul Carnell (Earth Resources Research 1983) 96 pages
Looks at the economic basis of intensive farming and the cost of alternative methods of meat and dairy production.

Ecology; Trees

The Death of Trees Nigel Dudley (Pluto 1985) 133 pages
A most interesting and informative account of the world situation regarding forests.

Sahara Conquest Richard St Barbe Baker

My Life, My Trees Richard St Barbe Baker (Findhorn Publications 1986) 188 pages

Who's Destroying the Forests: peasants or profits? The Ecologist vol. 12, no. 1 1982
The whole issue was given over to this topic.

Desertification Alan Grainger (Earthscan 1983) 96 pages
How people make deserts, how people can stop, and why they don't.

Natural Disasters: Acts of God or Acts of Man? Anders Wijkman and Lloyd Timberlake (Earthscan 1984) 126 pages

PERIODICALS

Ag-scene monthly £7 a year
From **Compassion in World Farming**

The Ecologist 6 issues a year £2 each, £12.50/year by post
From **The Ecologist, Worthyvale Manor Farm, Camelford, Cornwall PL32 9TT**

Hungry for Change newsletter
From **Oxfam**

Links quarterly £1.50
Magazine of **Third World First** A valuable source of information on, for example, colonialism (*issue 23*), transnational corporations (*issue 24, April 1986*)

New Ground 4 issues per year, 60p each
The Journal of Green Socialism from **SERA**

New Internationalist monthly 85p £11.70/year by post
From **42 Hythe Bridge Street, Oxford OX1 2EP**
Deals with world food problems, trade etc. and the relations between the rich and the poor.

New Leaves 4 issues a year 35p each
From the **Movement for Compassionate Living (The Vegan Way)**

New World bimonthly 30p
From **United Nations Association**

Oxfam News 4 issues a year
From **Oxfam**

Spur monthly 20p
From **World Development Movement**

The Vegan 4 issues per year 50p
From the **Vegan Society**

The Vegetarian bimonthly 65p
From some bookshops or from the **Vegetarian Society**

ORGANIZATIONS

Most of these organizations publish a range of books and leaflets. If writing for information or leaflets a stamped addressed envelope is appreciated.

Amnesty International (British Section)
5 Roberts Place, London EC1 0ES

Anti-Common Market Campaign
52 Fulham High Street, London SW6 3LQ

British Society for Social Responsibility in Science (BSSRS)
9 Poland Street, London W1V 3DG

Campaign Against the Arms Trade (CAAT)
11 Goodwin Street, London N4 3HQ

Campaign for Nuclear Disarmament (CND)
22-24 Underwood Street, London NI 7JG

Christian Aid
PO Box I, London SWIW 9BW

Compassion in World Farming (CIWF)
20 Lavant Street, Petersfield, Hants, GU32 3EW

Counter Information Services
9 Poland Street, London WIV 3DG

Earth Resources Research
258 Pentonville Road, London NI 9JY

Friends of the Earth (FoE)
377 City Road, London ECIV INA

Green Alliance
60 Chandos Place, London WC2N 4HG

Green Party
36/38 Clapham Road, London SW9 0JQ

Greenpeace
136 Graham Street, London NI 8LL

Henry Doubleday Research Association
National Centre for Organic Gardening, Ryton-on-Dunsmore, Coventry CV8

Minority Rights Group
29 Craven Street, London WC2N 5NT

Movement for Compassionate Living (The Vegan Way)
47 Highlands Road, Leatherhead, Surrey, KTII 8NG

Overseas Development Institute
10-11 Percy Street, London WIP 0JB

Oxfam
274 Banbury Road, Oxford, OX2 7DZ

Socialist Environment and Resources Association (SERA)
9 Poland Street, London, WIV 3DG

Third World First
232 Cowley Road, Oxford OX4 IUH

Traidcraft
Kingsway, Team Valley Trading Estate, Gateshead, Tyne and Wear NEII 0NE

United Nations Association
3 Whitehall Court, London SWIA 2EL

Vegan Society
33/35 George Street, Oxford OXI 2AY

Vegfam
'The Sanctuary' Lydford, near Okehampton, Devon EX20 4AL
Feeds the hungry without exploiting animals.

Vegetarian Society
Parkdale, Dunham Road, Altrincham, Cheshire WAI4 4QG

War on Want
I London Bridge Road, London SEI 9SG
World Development Movement (WDM)
Bedford Chambers, Covent Garden, London WC2E 3HA

Further details of most of these and many other organizations can be found in **Directory for the Environment** Michael J C Barker (Routledge & Kegan Paul 1986)

UNITS

I tonne = 1,000 kilograms = 2,205 pounds = 0.984 tons
I ton = 1.016 tonnes = 1,016 kilograms
I kilogram = 2.204 pounds   100 grammes = 3.527 ounces
I pound = 453.59 grammes   I ounce = 28.35 grammes

I hectare = 100 ares = 2.471 acres
I acre = 0.4047 hectares = 4,047 square metres
I square kilometre = 100 hectares = I million square metre
100 hectares = 0.386 square miles = 247 acres
I square mile = 640 acres = 259 hectares = 2.59 square kilometre
I are = I square decametre = 100 square metres = 119.6 sq. yards

I kilometre = 0.6214 miles (approximately ⅝ mile) = 1,093.6 yards
I mile = 1.609 kilometres = 1,609 metres
I inch = 2.54 centimetres = 25.4 millimetres
I metre = 100 centimetres = 1,000 millimetres = 39.37 inches

I litre = 1.76 pints   I pint = .568 litres

I Calorie (kilocalorie — often called a calorie) = 4.186 kilojoules
I kilojoule = 0.239 Calories

Compound interest growth

Rule to give approximate doubling period at r% (within range 0% to 10%):
divide 70 by r
for example: 4% per annum population increase:
doubling period = 70 ÷ 4 = 17½ years (error less than 1%)

ABBREVIATIONS

ACP	African, Caribbean and Pacific
BMA	British Medical Association
CAAT	Campaign against the Arms Trade
cal	calorie
CAMRA	Campaign for Real Ale
CAMREB	Campaign for Real Bread
CAP	Common Agricultural Policy
CBI	Confederation of British Industry
CIA	Central Intelligence Agency (USA)
EEC	European Economic Community (Common Market)
FAO	Food and Agriculture Organization (UN)
GNP	gross national product
HMSO	Her Majesty's Stationery Office
IBRD	International Bank for Reconstruction and Development (World Bank)
IBFAN	International Baby Foods Action Network
IDA	International Development Association
IFC	International Finance Corporation
IMF	International Monetary Fund
kg	kilogramme(s)
M	million
MAFF	Ministry of Agriculture, Fisheries and Food
MORI	Market and Opinion Research Institute
NATO	North Atlantic Treaty Organization
NEDC	National Economic Development Council
NEDO	National Economic Development Office
OPEC	Organization of Petroleum-Exporting Countries
TVP	textured vegetable protein
UK	United Kingdom
UN	United Nations
UNICEF	United Nations International Children's Emergency Fund — now United Nations Children's Fund
US	United States
USA	United States of America
USSR	Union of Soviet Socialist Republics
WDM	World Development Movement
WHO	World Health Organization (UN)

INDEX